joel ramirez

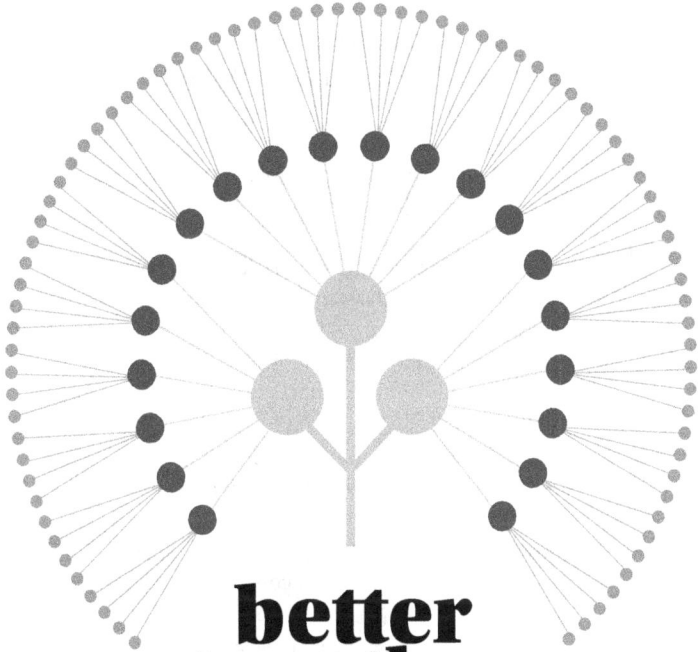

better together

why loneliness is killing us
and what we can do about it

Better Together

Why Loneliness Is Killing Us and What We Can Do About It

© Joel Ramirez, 2021
www.joelramirez.net
ISBN: 978-0-646-83011-7

Book cover design by Liz Knapp
www.mezzanine.co

Developmental editing by Allison Hiew
www.allison-hiew.squarespace.com

Copyediting by Lisa Ndeira
www.infowriteway.wixsite.com/writeway

Typesetting and layout by Julie Karen Hodgins
www.juliekaren.com

Printed by IngramSpark

This book is dedicated to my wife, Belinda,
my companion, my best friend. This book would not be
created without your loving support and unwavering
belief in me. My life is better together with you.

And to my children, Ruby and Logan. May you both
grow loving and caring for one another, and may you
have healthy relationships for the rest of your lives.

Table of Contents

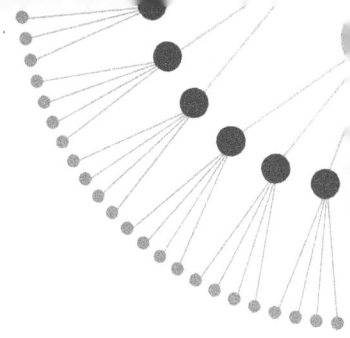

Foreword

BY GRAEME COWAN

I know first-hand how important caring and supportive relationships are to our wellbeing. When I went through a five-year episode of depression I withdrew from most of the people in my life. I felt ashamed that I could not cope. I thought I should be able to solve this problem myself. When I didn't have people to bounce my thoughts off, I found myself in an endless cycle of negative thinking.

I lost my job, my marriage broke down and I was unable to function. I thought my only option was to live with my parents. I was incredibly grateful for their support and I know now that I would not have made it without their unwavering love.

My recovery from depression was slow and there were many setbacks along the way. Regular daily exercise and meditation started my recovery and then I gradually started catching up with old friends and family, which helped immensely.

As my mood started to improve, I decided I wanted to write a book to share my and other people's stories of recovery. In *Back From the Brink,* I also shared the results of my survey of 4,064 people who had been through distressing times. I asked them what helped them most in their recovery. I wanted to explore most factors and asked respondents to rate specific medications, psychological interventions and lifestyle habits. This approach was never meant to provide a definitive answer about what treatment was best, but more to establish broad themes for a whole of person approach.

Respondents were asked to rate the treatments they had tried and how much they contributed to their recovery. Five major themes emerged.

- Emotional support and compassion
- Psychological treatments
- Lifestyle strategies
- Fulfilling work
- Prescription medication

Even if no magic bullet emerged for depression recovery, emotional support and compassion featured very strongly. This came from multiple sources including psychiatrists, psychologists, support groups, and family and friends.

Human care dominated the top ten most effective strategies.

These results emphasise what social creatures we are and how we crave empathy and connection. It was fascinating that the emotional support and reassurance from psychiatrists and psychologists were judged to be more important than the treatment they provided. This supports the medical literature, which shows that the quality of the relationship between the doctor/therapist and the patient is the best predictor of a successful outcome.

An especially important element of my sustained recovery was consciously rebuilding stronger relationships with people I liked and trusted, who I had withdrawn from. To build strong relationships, it is essential that being with the person is a positive experience, you see them regularly and you can be vulnerable with them.

When I reflect on my relationships pre-breakdown, these had the first two elements but not the third. Post-breakdown, I have worked hard to have four people in my life (plus my wife), that I can be vulnerable with. A problem shared is a problem halved.

Through my book, I met Gavin Larkin, the founder of R U OK? in March 2009. When he explained his plans of launching this movement later in the year, I knew I wanted to be involved. I was particularly attracted to the tagline: 'A conversation could change a life' because I knew through my own experience how important authentic conversations are to our mental health. It is incredibly rewarding to see how much R U OK? has grown in reach and impact.

Long-term studies also confirm how critical caring and supportive relationships are to a good life. The Harvard Grant study is the longest, beginning in 1938. It monitored the health and happiness of 238 Harvard sophomore students. They have been monitored every year for 80 plus years.

The current director of this study, Robert Waldinger, a professor of psychiatry at Harvard Medical School explains, "Taking care of your body is important, but tending to your relationships is a form of self-care too. That, I think, is the revelation".

Close relationships, more than money or fame, are what keep people happy throughout their lives, the study revealed. They are better predictors of long and happy lives than social class, IQ, or even genes. The key to healthy ageing is relationships, relationships and relationships.

This is why *Better Together* is such an important book. It is a real paradox in today's world that, despite being more connected via technology and social media than ever before, we find ourselves in a loneliness epidemic.

Recent research by APS and Swinburne University revealed that one in four (26.9 percent) Australian adults are lonely. When directly asked, using a one-item loneliness measure, one in two Australians (50.5 percent) reported feeling lonely at least one day in the previous week, while one in four (27.6 percent) reported feeling lonely for three or more days.

Through sharing his own story and other anecdotes, and a thorough literature review, Joel Ramirez reveals the benefits of close human connection. He explains why strong relationships make life worthwhile and are our scaffolding when things go wrong.

More importantly, Joel also explains the 'how' and 'what' of building these strong ties. May you strive for relationships that are mutually caring, supportive, and enjoyable. Who cares, wins.

GRAEME COWAN
Resilience speaker,
Author of book series *Back From the Brink*
and Board Director, R U OK?

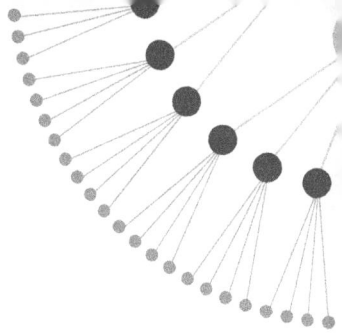

Introduction

WHY THIS BOOK; THIS TOPIC?

Before we begin, let me ask you some questions:

- Have you ever felt lonely?
- Have you felt lonely in the past month?
- Have you kept this feeling to yourself?
- Have you ever felt depressed as a result of loneliness?
- Do you know someone who might be feeling lonely?
- Have you ever felt alone in the workplace?

If you answered yes to one or more of these questions, I understand and I can relate. It's the reason I wrote *Better Together*.

After initially writing 70,000 words on the broader topic of mental health, I decided to rewrite the entire manuscript to focus on loneliness, social wellbeing and our need for human connection. Through the course of my interviews and research into the multifaceted causes of depression, I found that loneliness—specifically, the lack of meaningful relationships and social support in our lives—kept popping up as a key factor. Loneliness has the ability to greatly affect our wellbeing, how we interact with others and our life expectancy. It's something I couldn't deny the importance of any longer. I realised at that point that so much general awareness has been raised about mental health, but little to nothing on loneliness, which I would argue is one of the biggest and least addressed (or at least not taken seriously) public health issues today. My quest in this book has been to find out who is affected by loneliness, why it is happening, why it could actually kill us, then find and develop solutions to prevent loneliness from occurring in the first place. We can break the stigma around loneliness—together.

I was sitting in my friend's living room. Michael McQueen, a talented international speaker and prolific author, asked about what got me into writing on the topic of mental health.

I shared with him, "I went through chronic loneliness and depression after a really bad relationship breakup. I was in my early twenties at the time and realised I had no friends and no one to talk to. It felt like being in a big bubble, where I was shouting my lungs out, but no one could hear me. I would be surrounded by people yet still find myself crying out of nowhere. I felt completely alone in the world and there were times that I just wanted to end my life".

I then explained how moving to Sydney—where I found a job, and eventually started visiting a church and making new friends—was the best thing that could have happened as it helped me begin to combat my loneliness and overcome depression without needing to see a psychiatrist or start taking antidepressants. I know it's not everyone's story and I will be the first to suggest seeking professional help when needed; but, as I shared with Michael, things could have looked very different for me had I stayed in Melbourne and away from community.

"Coming to Sydney wasn't the final solution to my problems, but it was a circuit breaker. I couldn't dwell on my sorrows as much because this new city gave me new challenges and new experiences to focus my mind on. You know—work, learning to live on my own and finding myself. The real turning point was when I started meeting people again. Once I felt re-connected, I realised *that* was what I'd been longing for all along."

Thinking back on it, I went from feeling invisible to feeling like I belonged. For a long time, I couldn't understand why I'd become so sad and depressed when my girlfriend left me. I was a complete mess and I didn't know why I couldn't just pull myself together. But once I was in a good place and could think more clearly, I realised my worst fears had come true: I felt completely alone in the world. She was the only connection I had, and then it was gone.

Then I went to Sydney and *everything* changed.

Not knowing a single soul here at the time was a blessing in disguise. It was partly terrifying, yet exhilarating at the same time, because it gave me an overwhelming sense of freedom. More importantly, it enabled me to press the reset button to clear my mind and give me the space I needed to reinvent myself. I spent a lot of that first year soul-searching and understanding who I truly was. I used the time to observe the world and people around me, seeing new sights and places or going to cafés and restaurants by myself, even learning to play the guitar for the first time and immersing myself in my newfound talent. I enjoyed my own company for a while but, eventually, I longed for the company of others. After more than a year in Sydney, I was ready to make friends again, to reconnect again; but this time I knew who I was and the kind of people I wanted to attract into my life.

"I found myself coming to church by accident, where I met my first group of friends in Sydney. By 'accident', I mean I thought I was going to watch some band play at a place called Hillsong. I didn't know I was going to a church service!" I chuckled.

I then shared with Michael how I met some young adults there, similar ages to me, who accepted me for who I was and welcomed me with open arms. They introduced me to their friends, they invited me into their homes, and we got to do life together, and support and encourage one another. For the first time in a long time, I felt happy again.

As a result of the flourishing community around me, I began to flourish too: my mindset and outlook on life changed, my confidence levels grew; my thoughts and behaviour changed for the better. I thought, "Wow, this feels so good. I wish others could experience what I'm going through right now—this feeling of connectedness and belonging". It truly made me feel like I could achieve anything.

Eventually, I found coaches and mentors too, who were also in my ear guiding me through my personal and professional endeavours and, because of that, things changed for the better. That's not to say that life has become easy—I still go through many ups and downs with all the crazy challenges that life throws my way—but having these different circles of friends around me has certainly helped me to navigate and push through adversity.

As an aside, this isn't about me pushing for church specifically as a solution for everyone. What I *am* emphasising is the importance of building your personal community, and our need for a more connected society to help combat loneliness and its unwanted effects. It just so happens that a church community was the starting point and springboard which helped me to build my social and support networks.

"If I was to sum it all up, I realised that I can't possibly get through life alone. We are meant to do it *together*. So, if there's one thing I want to achieve from writing this book," I told Michael, "it's to share the power of connections and the importance of forming meaningful relationships".

"Joel, *that* is what your book is about!" Michael responded. "It's not about mental health, but about loneliness, about your story, about our need for connection. This will give you a focus point to talk about in the book. It's the right topic, at the right time, with you as the right person to write it because you've personally been through it."

My heart pounded a little when he said that. I had already written so much about mental health and dreaded the thought of rewriting my entire manuscript all over again. However, it was also the confirmation I needed to sharpen the focus of the book to a topic I had a very strong gut feeling about. Deep down, I really wanted to talk about loneliness as it was the common thread that kept popping up time and time again in my research.

My conversation with Michael is a case in point that we all need good friends (and coaches) to help steer us in the right direction. So, Michael, if you are reading this, thank you so much for your help and guidance. You are right: mental health is such a big, amorphous beast to tackle; but, with loneliness, not only do I now have a consistent and clear theme, but your feedback has helped me uncover what I believe is the biggest 'elephant in the room' on the topic of mental health.

To my readers, my objective is to share with you about the undesired effects of loneliness on our wellbeing—specifically, its devastating impacts on our physical health, our thoughts and behaviours when it becomes chronic; and its subsequent ripple effects on our relationships at home, at work and in our broader society. Ultimately, I want to explore what we can do about it.

I've read several books on the topic of loneliness and mental health, which were great for my research, but they were all written overseas in the UK and the US. This is why I wanted to localise the topic and write this book from an Australian's perspective. Like a journalist, my goal is to investigate, discover and share with you what's causing loneliness on our home soil, who experiences it, how to identify it in ourselves and others, and what we can do to combat and prevent loneliness from occurring in the first place.

In these chapters, I'll be sharing with you interviews I conducted with psychologists and local leading experts in the field, conversations with people on medication for their depression, and weaving in many other stories, including my own. Ultimately, I want to share with you *our* story and why *we,* as social beings, are *better together.*

One particular author I will be referencing from time to time in my book is the late John T. Cacioppo, who co-wrote a book called *Loneliness—Human Nature and the Need for Social Connection*, with William Patrick. Cacioppo was a professor of psychology, psychiatry and behavioural neuroscience, and founder and director of the Centre for Cognitive and Social Neuroscience at the University of Chicago. This man was the guru of scientific research on loneliness, with more than thirty years' experience. Sadly, Cacioppo passed away in 2018 at 66 years of age. I would love to have personally met and interviewed him for this book. Instead, I'll aim to refer to his knowledge and research where appropriate.

Finally, if you or someone you know may be feeling any signs of distress or mental health problems, then please browse through the references in the back of this book, which contain some useful website links and key contact numbers for emergencies.

Let's begin. ✤

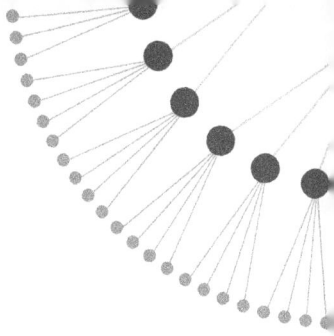

CHAPTER 1

A Contrast in Cultures

A CEO'S TRIP

Back in 2015, my CEO, John Munnelly, and I flew to the Philippines to launch our business in the local market there. At the time, we co-founded an online-based accounting software and, after a couple of years of running the business in Australia, we decided to test the solution out in another country to see how long it would take to build and sell the product there, then use that as a guide should we launch the software globally down the track. For various reasons, we decided to try it first in the Philippines, which is where I happen to have grown up before migrating to Australia with my family when I was ten years old.

The launch was a success. We had a huge turnout in Manila and I had the opportunity to address the crowd in their local language, tell them how proud I was to be a Filipino and to be launching this product in the Philippines with them. Cheekily, I then said, "Let's show the white man what we are capable of", as I pointed to John. I remember how the crowd went wild—they roared and cheered almost instantaneously. Suffice to say, my plan worked and I felt an immediate connection with them. They were my people.

On our flight back to Sydney, John and I sat next to one another and he congratulated me on my introduction. We went on to talk about business strategies in the Philippines when suddenly he interjected, "Those people [the Filipinos] don't have much but they seem happy. Why is that?"

John knew I was born there, so he wanted to understand my perspective and the context of the Filipino culture in relation to our two countries. I can understand how Westerners of wealthy nations, such as those who grew up here in Australia, can feel bemused by the insistent joy they see in poorer counterparts. After all, the Philippines, which has a population of more than one hundred million, has a poverty rate of about 26 percent. Manila, the city where John and I spent most of our business trip, has over *three million homeless people.* If you can imagine, that is almost 70 percent of the population of Sydney. Yet despite the rampant poverty, John was able to notice something different and positively unexpected about the country he observed and the people he came in contact with. Little did I know then that our conversation on the plane that day would become part of my book today.

"That's a good question", I replied. "You see, the Philippines may be economically poor but people there are rich in community. People back home [in Australia] may have lots of money and live in big houses but can still feel lonely in many ways. Sometimes we don't even know our neighbours. In a way, we're disconnected, and that's one of the differences between our two peoples."

"Yeah, wow," John responded contemplatively as he turned to gaze out through the tiny plane window next to him. I could tell he was processing what I had just explained to him. I can appreciate how what I'd said could sound so foreign to someone who grew up in Australia. However, being born and raised in the Philippines has given me the lived experience and insights to compare both cultures.

As I reflect on it, it is clear that close familial bonds and relationships are very important to Filipinos and often go beyond one's own bloodline to incorporate distant relatives and non-relatives alike, such as friends and neighbours.

I recall how people knew everyone in the neighbourhood and they'd share things with one another. When they cooked, they'd share what little food they had with their neighbours. Whenever there was a blackout, we would all go out onto the streets with our candlelight, where our parents would talk with friends and neighbours (ghost stories were always a special topic for Filipinos to share), while the kids listened or played together under the moonlight. When it rained, I remember running outside with my brothers, where we would play and dance in the downpour with the other kids. I can still smell that pleasant, earthy scent permeating the air like it was only yesterday.

Basketball also brings Filipinos together, in the same way football and cricket do for Australians. Every town had its own basketball court and everyone there would turn up to the local tournaments.

When there was a party, our neighbours would invite us, or we would invite them into our place. On special occasions, such as New Year's Eve, the entire neighbourhood would join in the midnight fireworks and celebrations on every street and corner, wishing each other a happy new year. I remember how this would continue for many hours, right through until the break of dawn. We lived for days like Christmas and New Year's Eve. The celebrations for the festive season would begin as early as September, as people would start to hang their decorations up everywhere and put up their Christmas trees. Life in the Philippines was and still is so full of struggles, so these celebrations helped people get by and set their worries aside.

The Filipinos have so much contact with their community that it brings them closer. It's like having one big extended family, so there's a very real and deep sense of belonging. They may not have much, but they are never alone. There is always someone you can talk to.

Things are a little bit different here in Australia and I am yet to experience the kind of connectedness and belonging the way I did back in the Philippines. As I sit here in my local library, in the leafy suburb of Lane Cove on Sydney's Lower North Shore, I look back at the almost thirty years I've lived in this beautiful country of ours. I'm reflecting on the many places I lived in, from the western suburbs of Melbourne to the eastern and northern suburbs of Sydney. I can honestly say that, for the most part, my experience has been the same across all locations, in that people go about their daily private lives without really getting to know the people in their neighbourhoods. Australians love their privacy. But I can only speak from my experiences living in these urban areas.

I do wonder what it's like in other parts of Australia. My developmental editor, Alison, told me how her husband was a dairy farmer in Southwest Victoria, where the community is quite cohesive and strong, thanks to football. During winter, she explained how it was almost all-consuming socially for those involved. It had good effects and negative ones as well, with the centrality of alcohol and the lack of other options if you weren't into footy. I heard many stories like hers about how country towns are small enough that people know everybody in the town. I wonder if it's anything like growing up in the Philippines. What do you think? Have you ever lived in a rural town? What was, or is, it like to live there?

Back in Sydney, in 2008, when I worked as a specialist executive recruiter, I found that half of the CEOs I met were divorced. When I asked what they would do differently if they had the chance, the response was always the same: "I would spend more quality time with my wife and kids". This insight had an impact on my life.

I can imagine a young man working hard to climb the corporate ladder or start his own business, then getting married, having kids, and buying that beautiful dream home. He then spends all his time working long hours and missing special events and memories with his children in order to maintain the lifestyle and pay the bills. Meanwhile, he and his spouse are growing apart. Eventually, they separate, and she takes the kids away with her. Now he's in his forties and all alone in this great big double-storey house with no one to talk to, not even his next-door neighbour who he's never really gotten to know, maybe aside from a brief chat in passing when they both take the bins out. He realises he does not have any close friends. Now he's wondering what life could have been like if only he was more present and spent more time with loved ones, and nurtured other important relationships as well. The thought of it all depresses him, so he's now seeing a psychologist so he can have someone to talk to and help him process his situation.

Unfortunately, this fictitious example is all too real in our urbanised society. We all either know someone who is going through something similar or can relate to this example personally. I can't help but think what kind of support this man could have had if only he were in the Philippines. Don't get me wrong, I love Australia and prefer living here for many reasons, but what if we could adopt some of the connectedness of the Philippines here in our own society … can you imagine the possibilities? I am convinced we would be happier, more resilient, and have a stronger nation for it.

So, what then are the reasons why Filipinos have such a tight-knit community, and what could we possibly learn from them to help combat the loneliness pandemic we are facing here in Australia? Luckily, I think I found just the man to help me answer this. ♣

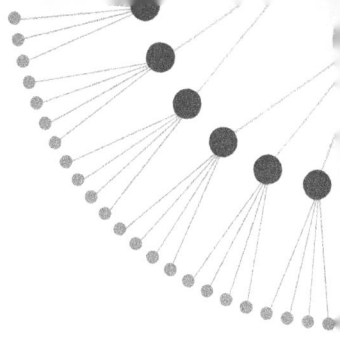

CHAPTER 2

The Effects of Shared Pain

A CLUE

I wanted to understand the reasons why Filipinos have such a tight-knit community. I had a hunch it was something to do with their shared economic struggles that helped them form such close bonds.

Looking back, I can't think of any close family or friends of mine in the Philippines who didn't go through poverty at some point in their lives, many of whom still struggle with it today. I remember how my friend's dad next door to us became unemployed and couldn't find work for many years, and how my mum used to share her home-cooked meals over the fence with them. We had so many neighbours like this who were jobless, many of whom constantly waited for money to arrive (such as from spouses or children overseas) just to survive. I learned how one of my cousins had died from a stomach ulcer, which was perhaps avoidable if he'd had access to the right nutrition and medical treatment. He simply dropped dead on the floor one day, leaving his young family behind. He never said anything about how he'd been feeling as he didn't want to burden anyone. He just endured the pain until it was too late. I was heartbroken—he was a kind human being. I would have paid for his doctor fees had I known. I remember giving him 500 dollars about a decade ago when he wanted to start a small piggery business, which he did but eventually had to shut down as he couldn't compete with the big leagues on price. I could keep writing tragic stories like this, but they would fill the entire book. My point is this: poverty is a real, big and ugly issue in the Philippines, but it also makes people more understanding, more aware of and more sympathetic toward one another in the process.

I wanted to find further evidence to help validate why, so I began searching online for clues, hoping to find an answer in a blog, discussion or study somewhere. My hunt brought me to an article entitled 'Shared Pain Brings People Together'[1] by the Association for Psychological Science. My eyes widened. *I knew it.*

The article explored how pain may actually have positive social consequences which foster cohesion—kind of like a social glue—within groups of people. More specifically, it referred to the work of Psychological Scientist and Lead Researcher Brock Bastian from the University of New South Wales, who was quoted as saying: "Our findings show that pain is a particularly powerful ingredient in producing bonding and cooperation between those who share painful experiences".

I thought, "*Wow, this is the guy I want to speak with*".

I typed Brock's name into Google and his academic profile popped up with an email address from the University of Melbourne. I quickly emailed him in excitement. I didn't know if his email would bounce. I didn't know if he would even read it or reply. But I remember telling him how much I enjoyed reading his research in the article, and how deeply it resonated with me. I explained how communities in the country where I came from formed solidarity through shared pain and how, through his research, I could finally validate why and how that would make them happier than the richest person in the world who lacked meaningful relationships in their life.

To my surprise, he emailed me back and was only too happy to meet at his office. It lined up perfectly with a work trip I had just booked to Melbourne so I told him I could catch up over lunch. He agreed, and we locked it in.

The day arrived and I went to meet Brock, now Associate Professor in the School of Psychological Sciences at Melbourne University.

It had been more than two decades since I last walked through the hallways and buildings of Melbourne University visiting one of my brothers, Francis, while he studied for his science degree. It was lunchtime and the walkways were littered with students holding textbooks and wearing university hoodies. For a moment, I felt young and free again.

I enjoyed walking amongst them as if I was about to go to my next class, but my suited attire reminded me that I was in a different life season now. As I walked the stairs and knocked on Brock's office door, I felt like I was 21 years old, a student coming to ask his professor about a project or an upcoming exam.

We decided to walk over to Lygon Street, famous for its Italian food and the place where Melbourne's café culture was born. We talked about life for a while, about family and kids, and his move across different states for work from Melbourne to Brisbane to Sydney and back to Melbourne again, where he landed his present job as an academic at the university. Finally, the conversation arrived at the topic of Brock's social experiments.

"In our first experiment, we assigned 54 students to submerge their hand into either painfully cold water or water that was room temperature, and we tasked them with locating metal balls in the water to place into a small container," said Brock.

In another experiment, the students either performed an upright wall squat, which is typically painful, or balanced on one leg where they could switch legs to avoid fatigue. He also described a third painful task, which involved eating spicy Bird's eye chili peppers.

The students were measured on how they felt about their group afterward and as it turned out, those who performed the painful tasks reported a greater degree of bonding than those who performed the painless tasks. Brock found that shared pain not only increased the group's solidarity but their cooperation as well. Those students who submerged their hands in the lukewarm water didn't end up engaging with one another; however, those who dipped their hands into painfully cold water had to use words of encouragement to help each other get through the task at hand. Brock explained that this enabled them to build stronger bonds with each other, and ultimately increase trust within the group.

I asked Brock about what inspired him to conduct the experiments, and he answered, "Do you remember the Queensland floods back in 2011? I was there at the time and I saw how the local people banded together to help those in need in the face of natural disaster. I thought, 'What if I could replicate this behaviour on a smaller scale using simple tasks in a controlled environment? Could we achieve similar results?'"

I remember seeing those devastating floods in Brisbane on television. Houses were completely submerged under water, entire suburbs going under, cars piled on top of each other, and people missing or found dead, all caused by powerful floods that wreaked havoc across Queensland. Anyone who saw it was completely shocked. I couldn't fathom how something like this could happen to our Sunshine State. It was the worst flood the state had experienced in over 35 years. But what amazed me even more than the flood itself were the 25,000 volunteers, dubbed the 'mud army', who all flowed into Brisbane with sleeves rolled up, lending their hands to complete strangers to help them get back on their feet. It was a 'faith-in-humanity-restored' kind of moment.

In both cases—the Queensland floods and Brock's social experiments—the element of shared pain was key, and it resulted in people bonding. Perhaps this is a clue as to why people in the Philippines have a special bond with their neighbours and the broader community. Their shared economic pain has, in the process, brought them closer together and acts as the 'social glue' I mentioned earlier, which binds them and keeps them *collectively* resilient—as a *group*—where they look out for one another, give words of encouragement, and show support through life's struggles. This makes me think about the important things in life, like friendship. Filipinos have a special community culture that is enviable. I certainly wouldn't mind having some of it here. I think we'd all feel less lonely and far happier.

Interestingly, in 2020 Australians began experiencing a nation-wide shared pain like no other—the COVID-19 Coronavirus pandemic. If people had never experienced loneliness or social isolation before, they had now. With lockdowns and physical distancing measures imposed across the country, you can see the kinds of economic impact and mental health breakdowns it's having on our society. Will this shared pain be enough to bring us and our communities closer together, and thus combat loneliness? I wish it were that simple but, unfortunately, there are other complicating factors at play in our culture that make it more challenging. I will go into these in the next chapter.

Another thing Brock said that stuck in my head was "we need some level of pain to be happy". In his book, *The Other Side of Happiness*, Brock states that we've become a culture addicted to positivity. We try to eradicate pain, we insulate ourselves and our children from risk and failure, yet the most thrilling moments of our lives have had elements of both pleasure and pain. Think of when you go for a run: it's not easy, you huff and puff, but after finishing you feel *great* about yourself. We call that feeling the 'runner's high'. Another example, which involves some of the deepest of pains, is giving birth. My wife, Belinda, endured twenty-one hours of excruciating labour pains, yet what followed next were feelings of indescribable joy and happiness as our firstborn arrived in the world.

How about when you start your own small business? It's stressful, it's challenging, and there's no guarantee of success. Yet it can also bring other rewards, such as the satisfaction of not having to work for someone else, and the respect you earn from your peers for having the courage to go out on your own. According to Brock, pain and hardship can increase our capacity for happiness. Think of the joy you feel after finishing exams or finally completing your degree. It feels good because you know the hard work you put into it. Nobody ever sees the extent of the pain you went through, but you got through it in the end. In all these examples, we become stronger, more resilient, and more connected to those we shared the journey with.

I had so many 'aha moments' during that short lunch break with Brock. I had never really linked pain to finding happiness until then, although I had always thought of pain and failure as something we grow and learn from. Brock's perspective, especially on shared pain and its positive social impacts, was eye-opening for me. It reminded me of the time Belinda and I took a CrossFit class when a friend invited us. Our group of first-timers had to complete a circuit in a certain amount of time, but I was completely exhausted after only two and a half minutes into a five-minute workout—I'd pushed myself too hard too soon. I remember dropping the medicine ball as I lay flat on the ground, unable to catch my breath. I felt like my heart was going to explode and I was ready to quit. Yet the group kept encouraging me to get back up, pushing me to complete the workout. "You can do it," one person said. "You've got this!" said another. By that point, others had also joined to encourage me to get back on my feet. It was what I needed to keep going and persevere. I couldn't have possibly mustered the energy to finish our timed workout without their support.

I learned something valuable that day more important than the workout itself: social support is a great motivator. What sets CrossFit apart from working out alone at a regular gym is its community culture. When you're worn out physically and mentally or you begin to doubt yourself, having encouraging people around helps you believe in yourself and pushes you to go further. We humans truly are *better together*.

As our meeting came to an end, Brock asked what I intended to do with my book.

"I'd like to use my book as a platform to reach out to people and break down the stigma around loneliness and depression. There are only so many hours in a day, so the book will allow me to reach and influence people I'll never get the time to meet," I explained.

I also told Brock that I wanted to localise the book and make it relevant for all Australians as many of the books published on mental health and loneliness have been written by authors overseas, with little insight provided about this great big land of ours. Though they were great for my research, I wanted to share stories and information provided by Australians for Australians, and my hope is that in the process, this book becomes more meaningful to you and your loved ones. ♣

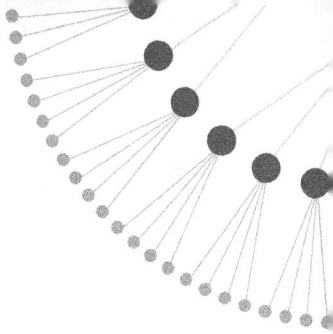

CHAPTER 3

Are Australians a Lonely Bunch?

I really wanted to know if Australia is a lonely country and if so, what's causing it. If having community and social support are important to our mental health and wellbeing, do we have these elements embedded in our culture? If we don't, why not?

At face value, Australia is considered one of the happiest countries in the world. According to 'The World Happiness Report'[1], three of the top 20 cities include Brisbane, Melbourne and Sydney. The report bases its findings on how happy each country's citizens perceive themselves to be and includes variables such as income, freedom, life expectancy, social support and generosity. I personally feel lucky to be in a country where it is predominantly safe, thanks in part to a government-initiated national gun buy-back program after Tasmania's Port Arthur massacre in 1996. Our geographical location has also kept us largely out of harm's way, reducing our exposure to serious agricultural diseases, political unrest and pandemics. In addition, our coastal areas are some of the most beautiful in the world, and citizens and travellers alike can choose their preferred climate zone from cold, snowy alpine regions in the south, to tropical weather and rainforests up north.

However, despite being surrounded by beauty and prosperity, the statistics on our sense of connectedness paint a very different picture, revealing that we are, in fact, a lonely nation. According to a 2016 Lifeline survey, two-thirds of 3,100 respondents said they "often felt lonely" and one-third indicated that they did not have someone to confide in when they felt lonely.[2]

'The Australian Loneliness Report'[3], produced by the Australian Psychological Society and Swinburne University, found that one in four respondents over the age of 18 were lonely. A closer look at the results provides some shocking insights into the most comprehensive study of loneliness completed in Australia. The survey asked questions such as how often you feel: "alone", "isolated from others", that "there is no one you can turn to", that you are "part of a group of friends", that "people are around you but not with you", and that "your relationships with others are not meaningful". A staggering 50 percent said they either always or sometimes felt alone. Interestingly, those aged over 65 were shown to be the least lonely, reporting better mental health and lower levels of social interaction anxiety than younger adults. In all, the report said that lonely Australians are 15.2 percent more likely to be depressed and 13.1 percent more likely to be anxious about social interactions than those who are not lonely. What did not come as a surprise was the result showing that lonely Australians have significantly worse physical and mental health, and poorer quality of life than their connected peers.

So, on one hand, 'The World Happiness Report' declares Australia to be one of the happiest nations in the world, but on the other hand, Lifeline reveals that many of us are still lonely despite living in this amazing country of ours. These findings leave me conflicted: how can we be truly happy if we are lonely? If we really are surrounded by such beauty and wealth, then what's causing our loneliness? I reached out to Clinical Psychologist and Senior Lecturer at Swinburne University, Dr Michelle Lim, to find out.

THE LONELINESS EXPERT

I learned of Michelle's work during my initial search for articles on loneliness when I came across one published by the ABC titled 'Feeling isolated? You're not alone. Here's why 1 in 4 of us is lonely'.[4] Michelle was quoted saying that chronic loneliness was on the rise in Australia and, as the Scientific Chair of the Australian Coalition to End Loneliness, both her words and her role caught my attention, so I quickly searched for her details and reached out via email. To my delight, she replied the following day and agreed to meet with me. I booked my flight to Melbourne and waited for the day with great anticipation. There were so many questions I wanted to ask, so much I wanted to learn from a local expert in the field.

Meeting Michelle actually began with a small challenge. She requested we meet at a local restaurant in Brunswick but when I arrived, it hadn't opened yet for the evening. I texted her to say it was closed so she picked me up in her car to search for a new destination together.

"I don't normally pick guys up like this, especially someone I don't know or have never met before," she said, and we both laughed. She then apologised for what she felt was a dirty car that hadn't been vacuumed for a while, adding, "Lucky you're not gonna write this part in your book, right?"

I said, "Yes, I will *absolutely* add this part to the book. It's what makes our story even better!" So, Michelle, if you're reading this, it's been shared with everyone now!

We connected instantly and talked in the car like we'd been friends for a long time. Michelle shared how her husband was also from the Philippines, and at that moment was stuck at Manila airport waiting for his flight back to Australia. It was an easy starting place, talking all things Filipino, including places we'd both been to and local dishes Michelle loves.

When we arrived at the bar and ordered wine, I asked Michelle about her story and how she came to research loneliness.

"I was the first person in my family to go to university," said Michelle. "In 2011 I went to live in the US for a couple of years with my husband to do my post-doctoral research and I happened to be measuring loneliness and social anxiety at Washington University. I remember there was a tornado one time while I was on the phone with my friend when suddenly our connection was cut off and I could no longer talk with her. Even though my husband was there, I felt lonely and isolated being so far away from home [in Melbourne]. I wanted to speak with my friend. I *needed* her."

Hearing Michelle say this at the time reminded me that we are all human: even trained clinical psychologists can feel lonely. It's not that her husband wasn't enough, it's just that sometimes we all need to be surrounded by friends. Unfortunately for Michelle, her closest friends and family were back home in Australia.

A friend of mine, Matt, had a somewhat similar experience when he got married and travelled through South America with his wife for six months. It was going well for a while but eventually, they grew impatient with each other, sometimes arguing about the smallest things. I asked Matt what they argued about and he said, "I don't know, really. It's embarrassing. Sometimes we just had to sit away from each other on the bus and give each other space. I think spending 24 hours a day with the same person every single day isn't good for you". Although their scenarios were different, it made me think how two years away from home would make Michelle really miss her friends. It isn't sustainable to depend on a single person to fulfil all our relationship needs.

When Michelle returned to Australia, a woman by the name of Lesley, who previously worked as chief finance officer of Relationships Australia, reached out to her.

"Lesley told me she knew people in the not-for-profit sector, and I knew people in academia. 'Why don't we team up and start a coalition to end loneliness?'" Michelle relayed to me. "We identified that it's a big issue in Australia. That was three years ago now [2016] and we've been raising awareness of and addressing loneliness and physical isolation through evidence-based interventions and advocacy since that time. Our plan is to be the peak body for loneliness."

After listening to her story, I still had one unanswered question I was desperate to ask Michelle: "So *why* are we lonely?" I didn't know what answer to expect. I had some ideas, but her swift response blew my mind.

"Oh, that's easy," said Michelle. "We're too wealthy."

"Huh?" I replied, puzzled. "What do you mean? That's it?"

"Think about it. When we're wealthy, we don't need help and support from people. The people in the Philippines require groups, which acts as a protective factor. Over there you would typically be okay because the community takes care of the individual."

Reflecting on my own childhood experience, I know this to be true. In the Philippines, the community is tight-knit, and often comprises a combination of family, friends and other people who live in the neighbourhood. Imagine how comforting it would be when you're having a bad day if you could simply call on your neighbours for help or support. In retrospect, I find it's quite uncommon to have this sense of belonging and friendship with neighbours here in Australia. Occasionally, I hear about some streets here and there where neighbours get along well, but it's more the exception rather than the rule. When I look outside my front window here in Sydney, I see a row of houses before me, but sadly I don't think I've ever met or spoken with anyone from those homes. Most people are private and keep to themselves.

Fortunately for us, Belinda and I befriended the people in our own apartment building who we can rely on for support and community when needed, but we had to be intentional in building those relationships. To our delight, sometimes we'd be surprised with how neighbourly some people can be. I remember the day after we arrived home from hospital with our newborn son, Logan, and there in front of our door was a shopping bag containing bread, milk and fruit, left there by an anonymous neighbour. We later discovered it was from a young couple upstairs who we'd not yet met—Bruce and Olivia—who, a couple of months earlier, had given birth to a child of their own. They knew we'd just arrived home and all too well what it felt like to have a newborn, so didn't want us to have to worry about buying food that day. The blessing went beyond simply having food on the table for a day: we formed a special bond, with our two families often spending time together, even in passing as our two boys knock on one another's front doors to simply say hello. We trusted one another with our spare keys and would frequently exchange dinner ingredients, a glass of wine or a scoop of ice cream. What I learned from Bruce and Olivia is that building community and friendships starts and grows with intentionality. If you truly want to know your neighbour you *have* to make the first step.

Michelle's perspective on Australians being "too wealthy" for our own good ties in well with my earlier conversation with Brock Bastian, who found that shared pain brings people together. It makes absolute sense to me now, how the economic struggles in the Philippines bring people closer together. They need each other to survive. People who have money, however, are less likely to reach out for help, and when you don't ask for help, you don't get help, and the net effect is fewer meaningful bonds and connections made with the people in your community. Being wealthy is like wishing to be rich from a genie in a bottle: there's a catch. You can be wealthy, but chances are you'll also be lonely. Ironically, it seems Australians are lonely together.

OUR CULTURE

In addition to the conundrum of too much wealth and too little pain, I wanted to look deeper into Australian cultural values to understand what else is contributing to our loneliness.

During my research, I came across Hofstede Insights, a Dutch organisation that enables people to solve inter-cultural and organisational culture challenges around the world. Their insights provided me with an understanding of Australian culture that I'd never really considered before. One in particular that caught my attention was that we are a highly individualistic culture, scoring 90 out of 100 on Hofstede's Individualism Scale.[5] According to the company, this means Australians are "a loosely-knit society in which the expectation is that people look after themselves and their immediate families". Could this priority of 'me' over 'we' be one of the causes behind loneliness in our society?

The opposite of an individualist nation is a collective one, where the needs and goals of the group take priority above self. The Philippines is a classic example, sitting at 32 out of 100 on the Individualism Scale, which makes them largely collectivist in nature. This collectivism is seen most clearly in overseas Filipino workers, who regularly transfer a large portion of their earnings to their loved ones back home. As the main, and often only source of income in the family, these workers remit money, which becomes vital support for dependent family members, including spouses, children, siblings and parents. In some cases, their large extended families benefit as well. By contrast, when I think about Australian culture, we gladly look after our immediate family— that is, our partner and kids (and sometimes our parents)— but often hesitate to extend our wealth beyond that.

So, what are the implications and correlations with respect to loneliness in Australia, considering we came in at 90 out of 100 on the Individualism Scale? Wanting to learn more about the story behind these numbers, I looked for someone to speak with at Hofstede Insights. To my delight and good fortune, I found David Morley, the managing director of Hofstede Insights Australia. I caught up with David in Sydney to find out more.

David looked like an absolute boss in his fifties. He was tall and confident in his long-sleeved shirt and sports jacket but had a sense of warmth and kindness about him also. As soon as he saw me, he smiled and said, "Hey man, it's really great to meet you," and shook my hand. I could tell that David, as a culture expert, was already working on relating with me, an approach I appreciated, considering it was I who asked for help, not the other way around.

I took David to a local café in North Sydney's business district and we sat down over coffee. We briefly spoke of each other's journey but regrettably didn't have much time together, so we saved the 'getting to know each other' conversation for another day.

"David, I'm fascinated about your work at Hofstede Insights and what your team does," I said to him. "How did it all begin?"

"Well, our Founder and Social Psychologist, Geert Hofstede, had access to IBM as a former employee. Back in the sixties, IBM was one of the few organisations with a large number of culturally diverse employees globally. Luckily for us, they were open to Geert's research, which validated his theory on cultural values, including individualism versus collectivism, and masculinity versus femininity, among others. It wasn't until the nineties that we then introduced short-term versus long-term oriented countries into our cultural dimensions. For example, countries like Japan are long-term focused. Panasonic had a 150-year plan, would you believe? Anglo countries, on the other hand, are short-term oriented, so a five-year business plan is already long. All of these cultural values have a part to play in your research on loneliness."

"Yeah, right," I replied pensively. "Can we dig into that a bit further? In regards to loneliness, I'm trying to find the link between that and us Aussies who form an individualistic society, as opposed to collectivistic nations such as my home country, the Philippines. Can you tell me your thoughts on that, please?"

"Sure," David said, leaning in. "In Australia, it's more than just the individual piece. Let me start by saying that people in collectivist countries can be lonely, too, for different reasons. In an individualistic society, it's about autonomy: what *I* think is important. People set personal goals and objectives based on the self: it's about me, not we. In a collective society, it's about family: people are motivated by the group's goals, what is best for the collective group and belonging. Loneliness comes when your sense of belonging is driven by what other people think and how they dictate what it means to belong. It's a catch-22 almost. In Australia, the culture is 'I'll look after myself. I'll figure it out. It's okay for me to be me and to go out there and select my own group of friends'. There's a relative amount of comfort in that. But it's when we can't find that confidant that it gets tough."

David paused before continuing.

"Australia is also a masculine society where it's about being the best and being associated with the best. This can make us single-minded around what we think is right. In a masculine culture, men, in particular, are expected to be competitive, assertive and focused on material success. By contrast, in a feminine society, men and women are both expected to be more nurturing and focused on people and quality of life. On top of that, we're also short-term oriented where our horizon is right there," David said as he placed his right hand a short distance in front of him.

"For example, in business, we don't give ourselves time to develop relationships. We have to get straight down to business." It was at this point I told him how ironic it was that we went straight to business talk as he just described, but David was understanding—he knew we didn't have a lot of time and simply wanted to impart as much insight as he possibly could.

"In a collectivist nation, trust is built on who I know you are. When an Anglo goes to Asia, they go straight to business. Meanwhile, in Chinese culture, for example, they want to go out for meals first, but the Anglo wants to get on task and get it done. Also, when you go to a collectivist country, it's about the group and harmony. Being singled out and honoured as an individual from the rest of the team may be embarrassing for that person. There was this expat I knew who was dropped into Beijing. I was his coach. As soon as he was parachuted in, he quickly pointed out that nobody there got recognised for their work and that his plan was to start showing recognition to individuals who did a great job. I quickly told him no, that it's a bad strategy. You can't think like that in a collectivist society who wants to belong." David described it from a collectivist viewpoint, "Placing me above the group is like shaming me in front of the group. Over there, the group wins, not the individual".

"Coming back to loneliness, our short-term horizon is here." David placed his hand again in front of him. "From that point of view, people need to fit in with us. We are nationalist-type thinkers. So, if you're an immigrant in this country for example, where English is not your first language, it is going to be very difficult to fit in. With Australians being short-term oriented, they don't have the patience to wait for you to start speaking their language. It's just too hard. They'd rather move on. If you come from overseas and you look different, you don't fit. The ones who do survive are the ones who show they fit in. Unfortunately, the only saving grace is if you come from other white nations, you at least have the advantage because you look the same until you open your mouth. It's sad, but it's our reality."

As I reflect on what David said, I think of the time I moved to Australia with my family and how difficult it was for us to fit in as new immigrants. I won't go into detail about it here, as I talk more about it in a later chapter, but based on what we experienced, I do wish there was a way Australians could be more long-term oriented. Perhaps then as a nation, we would be more patient, giving others time to catch up with our language and culture, even taking the time to walk the journey together.

Even as I recall the hardships we faced as migrants, I'm encouraged by Michelle's words during our conversation:

"Joel, what you're doing adds immense value. You've got it from a first-person perspective. Talk about your journey because that's really relatable. Talk about it from a minority perspective. You have an opportunity to educate people who aren't part of the minority and explain to them the barriers you had to overcome and how you had to work harder than everyone else to get there. I too believe that creating this awareness piece is an important first step toward bringing our people together". Thanks for the encouragement, Michelle.

My meeting with David ended on the hour, but I knew we would meet again. His insight and knowledge into different cultures captivated me. I came to see him to find out if there was a correlation between loneliness and individualism. Instead, he gave me more than what I bargained for: we've now learned that our tendency towards individualism, *as well as* masculinity and short-term orientation, are more than likely contributing to our loneliness epidemic in Australia. After meeting with David, I believe now more than ever that our relationships would improve if only we had a better understanding of one another's diverse nationalities, backgrounds, faiths, values and beliefs. Maybe we would have fewer cases of loneliness as we become more accepting and more understanding. Perhaps a sprinkle of that collectivist mindset wouldn't hurt us either. As an individualist nation, we often try to solve things on our own, we try to make it on our own. If there's anything I've learned so far, it's that asking for help and support can be a good thing, which deepens our relationships with others in the process. ✣

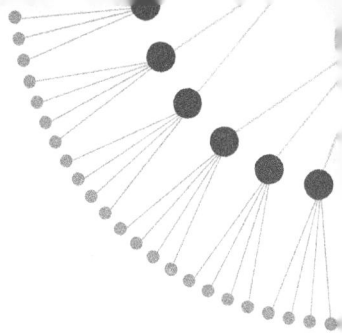

CHAPTER 4

What Happens When We Feel Lonely?

As humans, we can't survive long in isolation. It is important that we have social contact. I remember watching a social isolation experiment on TV many years ago. The volunteer's mission was to stay in an apartment for about a week with no television, phone or radio, and he was not allowed any contact with the outside world. There were cameras installed in all the rooms so you could observe and listen to what he was up to. At first, the volunteer thought he could handle it, and so the first couple of days went by without a hitch. He smiled and spoke to the camcorder, played the guitar, exercised, took long showers, ate and had a good night's sleep. By mid-week, however, his behaviour began to change. He became restless, unable to relax, pacing back and forth from here to there. The boredom and deprivation of interactions were making him anxious, and he was speaking less to the camera. By the end of the week, he *finally* cracked and declared he'd had enough. He threw a chair across the room and refused to speak in front of the camcorder altogether. When the experiment ended, the volunteer opened the door and walked himself out onto the busy street filled with people. I remember him explaining how happy he was, how he enjoyed seeing people's faces, how he appreciated looking at the trees, flowers and his surroundings—things he once took for granted. He was breathing it all in and looked to be in a state of euphoria.

What this experiment taught me is that we are ultimately relational creatures, in need of contact with others and nature to function well and stay happy (not just food and a place to rest). The experiment may have lasted for only a short period of time, but it'd already had a negative impact on the volunteer's wellbeing. Can you imagine what it would be like if you were to live in isolation like that, week after week, year after year, with minimal social contact—no circle of friends, nor community? I don't know about you, but I wouldn't be able to stay sane for long.

DEFINING LONELINESS

According to Collins Dictionary, "Loneliness is the unhappiness that is felt by someone because they do not have any friends or do not have anyone to talk to".[1] I don't believe this definition encompasses the full meaning of the word.

To me, loneliness is a little more complex than that. As we learned from Dr Michelle Lim, she felt lonely being away from family and friends when she did her PhD in the US. It wasn't for the lack of friends or anyone to talk to. She had her husband and work colleagues to talk to, but her feeling of loneliness was amplified by being geographically distant from people she had deep connections with.

This reminds me of the time I attended a Microsoft conference in Florida in the US several years ago. The software company I co-founded was built in partnership with Microsoft, and each year the software giant would host the largest IT conference on the planet. Thousands of partners from all over the globe would fly to the States for a week-long event to learn, be inspired, connect with other partners, and have the opportunity to brush shoulders with senior leadership from Microsoft HQ. It was 2018 and Microsoft was throwing a massive end-of-conference party at Disney World for their global partners. At first, I was over the moon. I remember telling my wife how I had always wanted to go to Disneyland, ever since I was a kid. Unfortunately, I ended up going by myself as my colleague had to stay back with some people from Microsoft but agreed to rendezvous at some point at the theme park. I remember hopping on one of the many coaches Microsoft had hired, but when I looked around, I found myself surrounded by unfamiliar faces. I didn't mind at first—I supposed as delegates we were all in the same boat, converging from various parts of the world, and the little boy in me was still filled with excitement and anticipation—I was finally going to Disney

World. But as we arrived, I noticed people coming in pairs with a friend or colleague, some had even brought their families along with them, while I was on my own. I found myself walking around the park alone, which wasn't fun at all. I was surrounded by people, yet I had no one to share this once-in-a-lifetime experience with. Instead, I felt miserable and, for the first time on that business trip, I wanted to come home. I couldn't wait to get out of there and back to the hotel, so I hopped back on an almost empty bus and left.

So, what happened to me?

Lifeline.org.au says that "Loneliness is a feeling of sadness or distress about being by yourself or feeling disconnected from the world around you".[2] This describes what I felt at Disney World. What should have been a great time was washed out with feelings of sadness and disconnectedness. What I needed was to share that experience in the company of friends or family but, like Michelle, I was a long way from home.

Although Lifeline has a more accurate definition of loneliness than Collins dictionary, I still don't think it completely captures the full extent of loneliness. What I have come to realise is that loneliness isn't simply the absence of people, but it extends to the absence, distancing, or loss of deep and meaningful relationships.

So, how does this definition play out?

Someone may live in solitude and not have a whole lot of contact with others, but enough meaningful connections to not experience feelings of loneliness, even if others perceive them to be socially isolated. On the flip side, an individual might be surrounded by people and appear socially engaged, yet still not feel like they belong or that they're part of the group. Hence, feelings of loneliness may be more closely linked to the *quality* of relationships one has, not just the quantity. This helps to explain why I used to feel like crying when I was experiencing depression, whether I was in a busy shopping centre filled with people or at birthday parties I was invited to. Deep down I was feeling very lonely and utterly miserable.

So, what exactly was going on inside my mind and body?

Michelle explained during our catch-up that loneliness is akin to hunger and thirst. When you're hungry, you eat. When you're thirsty, you drink. In other words, when you're feeling lonely, Michelle said, "Your body is asking you to reach out. It's telling you that your connections (or lack thereof) are not good enough. Loneliness protects us this way as it highlights our need for social connections. You can't change thousands of years of algorithms. It's there to help you survive".

I was mind-blown after she said that. Who would have thought that feeling lonely could be beneficial? Yet Michelle's words make absolute sense. However, unlike thirst or hunger, which may be satisfied with food or water, loneliness requires an authentic interaction between *two* people—not as easy a task. To compound this, the other person needs to reciprocate the same level of intimacy in the conversation for it to be meaningful.

I further learned from Michelle that loneliness can be acute but can also become chronic. What happened to me in Disney World was a short-term bout of loneliness. It was mild and brief and could happen to anyone at some point in their life. In fact, transient loneliness is so common that we accept it as part of day-to-day life. *Chronic* loneliness happens when the feelings of loneliness or isolation continue long term and begin to impact many areas of our lives. I asked Michelle what we could do to solve loneliness, and although a forthright solution eluded our conversation, she affirmed, "Acute loneliness is okay—as I mentioned, it reminds us to reach out—but we must absolutely solve chronic loneliness".

But *why* do we need to solve chronic loneliness? According to John T. Cacioppo, author of *Loneliness—Human Nature and the Need for Social Connection*, loneliness becomes an issue when it "creates a persistent, self-reinforcing loop of negative thoughts, sensations and behaviours".[3] As it turns out, over time, feelings of disconnection significantly influence our minds, bodies and behaviours, and can have some pretty devastating effects when they become chronic. I am going to refer to many of Cacioppo's research findings in this chapter to explain what those effects are; but, in the meantime, let me share my own story of how loneliness affected my life.

❖ ❖ ❖

In my early twenties, I suffered greatly from chronic loneliness, which led to my depression and ultimately, suicidal thoughts. I had been dating a girl who, after four years together, decided to call it quits and broke up with me.

That day was the beginning of my mental health breakdown.

When she left me, I realised I had no one to turn to, no network of support, and I certainly couldn't handle it on my own. It took me months before I could even say anything to my parents, and I was too ashamed to say anything at all to my two brothers. Even if I wanted to speak up, I didn't know how, and to make matters worse I had no close friends to confide in because I hadn't bothered nurturing the few friendships I did have before and during the relationship. I lost count of the times my friends told me they were losing me. I simply laughed them off and carried on focusing all of my energy on this one individual. By the time my girlfriend and I separated, I could no longer reach out to my old friends. I couldn't bring myself to do it. Surely they wouldn't want me back or to hear from me again, I reasoned. What if they argued that the only reason I was calling was because of the breakup? What would I say? The truth was they would have been entirely correct.

The thought of having no girlfriend and no friends was devastating. Thinking I was now alone in the world and completely isolated paralysed me from head to toe. People say when you're going through a rough patch that it gets easier as time goes by, but that wasn't the case for me at all. If anything, it felt like I was sinking deeper and deeper into the ocean.

Sometimes I would get panic attacks and not be able to breathe. I remember one of those moments quite vividly. I was on the train one day on my way to university in the city, where I was studying IT. I hopped on a carriage at Laverton station and sat down with a heavy heart, thinking about my life and an uncertain, miserable future ahead of me. All of a sudden, I started weeping. There were people around me—the carriage was about a third full—but I couldn't control my emotions. I looked out the window to try to distract my thoughts, but the feeling was overwhelming. I tried to sob as quietly as possible, my hands trembling as I held on to keep my mouth shut. "Isn't anyone out there who can help me?" I screamed silently, pleading in my head. The thought of being alone with no shoulder to cry on was crushing. I began to hyperventilate, unable to control my rapid breathing. It was so bad that it felt like I had a bag over my head, choking and suffocating me. I held on to my neck as I desperately gasped for air. I looked out the window once more at the passing tracks, and eventually calmed myself down and began to breathe normally again. That feeling of breathlessness was probably one of the most terrifying experiences I've ever had; but, sadly, I was about to face many other difficult challenges that year.

First, I lost focus on my part-time studies and began failing some of my subjects at university. Next, my boss was a bully at the domain and website hosting internet company I was working for. He never made me feel acknowledged or valued, and he said things behind my back, and other people's backs, too. Thirdly, and possibly the most traumatic, I had two major car accidents. It was a triple whammy, each blow more devastating than the last.

In my first car accident, I was on the Westgate Bridge travelling 80 kilometres per hour, when the front bumper of the truck ahead of me fell underneath it, with the tyres catapulting the entire piece of metal straight for my head. Luckily, I swerved, and it struck my right window frame instead, completely bending it in, and missing my face by centimetres. According to the policeman inspecting the crash, had I not moved the steering wheel in that split second, I could have died instantly.

In the second accident, I had been attempting to make a U-turn when I was suddenly t-boned by an oncoming car, spinning my car around. Clearly, I'd misjudged the distance and speed of the other driver. To me, he'd looked far enough away to take my turn. Was my mind somewhere else? Was my perspective hazed by something? Thankfully, he was okay and even got out to check if I was alright. I was, but also completely dazed and confused as to how it had all just happened in the blink of an eye. I was without a car for several months after that accident. No car meant no freedom: no getting in any time I wanted to, driving wherever I wanted to. Without my car, it felt like I'd lost the only thing that made me feel like I was in control. Being home all the time, my parents tried their best to invite me along to their social events, but I couldn't force myself to go. I found myself not wanting to leave the house anymore. There were times when I couldn't even get myself out of bed. When you're going through depression, sometimes you just feel like there is nothing to look forward to anymore.

The year that followed was just as difficult, if not harder. I became an insomniac, forced to listen to an endless chatter of negative thoughts streaming through my mind every time I went to bed. I was constantly sleep-deprived, so I started taking sleeping tablets, which worked for a while until eventually, their effects stopped altogether. It was so frustrating. On one occasion, I found myself staying awake for more than 48 hours. I was beyond exhausted. I became so desperate that I took the last two sleeping tablets I could find, and—against all reason—took six paracetamol tablets with it. You aren't meant to combine the two drugs, let alone overdose on one. I'd only hoped that maybe I'd finally get some of the sleep that kept evading me. How wrong I was. Instead, it wasn't long until I started vomiting, feeling dizzy, and getting a killer headache in the process, but *still* no sleep. My desperate situation went from bad to worse, and I vowed never to try it again.

When sleep finally did greet me, things didn't get any better. Something new and frightening began to happen. I started having recurring nightmares of being chased down by bad people or, more disturbingly, dreams of out-of-body experiences where I would wake up and stare at myself from above. I would then find myself waking up with sleep paralysis, unable to move. It was as if my body, hands and feet were being pressed down against my will and there was nothing I could do about it. It was a terrifying thing to experience. Now I had a dilemma: on one hand, I desperately wanted to get some sleep; but on the other, I was afraid of what would happen if I did.

If that wasn't enough, I was also beginning to see things that shouldn't be happening: objects would be moved by an invisible hand—a stuffed toy I'd won at a carnival would suddenly fly across the room. At other times, I would see a translucent life-like form, a barely visible shape standing in front of me. Was I hallucinating as a result of my depression and major sleep deprivation? Was it something more sinister? Either way, I couldn't tell you what was real or pure imagination. I remember confiding in my dad about these experiences and telling him that perhaps I was going crazy. I said that I thought I should see someone about it but he didn't know what to do himself, so he simply told me to rest and to try to get some sleep. Looking back, I think he was probably out of his depth and not equipped to deal with my mental health problems, so he wasn't able to give me the advice I needed at the time. But I don't blame him at all for that—he was so caring and supportive during my darkest moments. Back in the nineties and early 2000s, there was simply a lack of awareness campaigns around depression and mental health the way we have today. I'm sure many other parents would have been in the same boat as mine, not knowing what to say or do in the same situation. At the time, the most heavily promoted safety ads we saw on TV were about the risks of smoking and drink-driving, but there was nothing on mental health. Today, the topic of wellbeing has taken its rightful place at the forefront of media and mainstream society. We even have buses completely plastered with 'RU OK?' signage. There are so many resources to take up and places to go for help. In fact, I'm going to pause here and implore you: if you or someone you know might be experiencing hallucinations similar to what I have just described, please seek for yourself or encourage your loved one to go to see a professional. I have provided some points of contact in the back of this book as a starting place—flick to it now and take the first step. *Don't* allow your wellbeing to deteriorate without seeking medical attention as I did, because things only got worse for me: one day, I contemplated taking my own life.

I'd had suicidal thoughts before, but somehow this time I wanted to do it for real. I was home alone one day in our house in Altona Meadows, and I could see the garage in front of me. I began to wonder if there was a rope inside that I could somehow tie into a noose. I closed my eyes and imagined placing the rope around my neck and proceeding to hang myself from the roof beam. Suddenly, I could feel the hairs stand up over my entire body. All I could see and feel at that point was darkness, enveloping me like it was some kind of entity pressing me to go ahead and do it. I opened my eyes and had a vision of my parents outside the garage, watching my now lifeless body, Dad trying to lift Mum off the ground, who was screaming and weeping in agony. I looked at them both and thought, "Why are you guys crying? It's over now. My pain is gone. I'm set free".

My phone rang, snapping me back to reality like a bungee cord.

"Hello, is this Mr Ramirez?" the man asked.

"Yes," I replied flatly.

"Ah, great! My name is Ian, and I'm currently recruiting for a fast-growing business here in Sydney, which competes with your current employer. You were referred to us by a colleague of yours and we'd like to make you an offer to work for an up-and-coming web hosting company," he explained. Ian went on to describe how the role required me to relocate interstate and was similar to what I had been doing but at twice the salary and with perks like paid rental allowance and paid flights back to Melbourne so I could visit my family once a month. It was a very enticing deal, but my mind was still in a daze from being snatched from the cliff's edge of suicide I'd been walking along only moments earlier.

His blur of job details had suddenly halted. "What do you think, Joel?"

"Hey, uh, I'm kind of busy at the moment. Can you ring back some other time?" I answered dazedly. I must have sounded disinterested.

"Oh, did you hear the offer I just mentioned?" he asked, puzzled. It was an opportunity of a lifetime but having just been in the middle of seriously contemplating suicide, I wasn't in the mood to talk about jobs, salaries or relocating to another state.

"Yes. Let me think it through," I replied. We exchanged details and I hung up.

That call saved my life. It was impeccable timing, the perfect interruption to those dark thoughts running through my head. When the call ended, I began to think about my parents, and how taking my own life would have left an unspeakable amount of pain and sorrow behind. I don't know how the vision of my parents weeping on the floor came to mind, but it crystalised for me just how important I must have been to them.

When they came home that day and Dad opened the door, I remember falling into their arms and weeping like a child, like I'd never wept before. I told them how lonely I'd been feeling, how I wished I'd reached out to them sooner, and how I wished I could be happy again. I didn't know what the word 'depression' meant at the time, so all I could say was how deeply sad I was and how excruciatingly painful the feeling was. Without judgement, my parents told me how much they loved me and how they understood that what I was going through must have been very difficult. They gently cradled me in their arms like a parent to a small boy. I didn't want it to end. It's amazing what a simple touch or embrace can do, how it makes you feel comforted and loved, and how powerfully it heals your soul. Opening up to my parents that day was such a release, like a burden now shared that I wouldn't have to bear alone anymore. Reconnecting with them that day pulled me back from the brink. Ma and Pa, when you read this, thank you. You don't understand how much you helped me that day. Your simple actions were a giant first step in my recovery.

On a side note, hugging releases the chemical oxytocin, which reduces stress and blood pressure, and gives you a whole range of positive moods and emotions.[4] This is why many call it 'the love hormone' and it makes perfect sense as to why I wanted to stay for so long in my parents' embrace.

By the way, I took the job—thank you, Ian. It was a decision that changed my life forever. What I do know is that I wasn't meant to die then, I wasn't meant to cut my life short. I am meant to be right here, writing this book, to let you and others know you are not alone.

I understand first-hand, and at such an intimate level, what Michelle meant when she said that we must absolutely solve chronic loneliness. It is debilitating and can have utterly devastating effects. In my case, it led to depression. And in some unfortunate cases, it can even lead people to take their own lives. It almost took mine.

WHAT THE EVIDENCE TELLS US

Having experienced first-hand what it looks and feels like to be chronically lonely, I was curious to understand what others have discovered about its devastating effects.

ON BEHAVIOURS

According to Cacioppo, as loneliness persists, we start to lose our ability to self-regulate, which is a critical building block of resilience. Successful self-regulation depends on our ability to cope with challenges—not just by appearing well-balanced or self-controlled but actually feeling it deep within ourselves[5]. This ability to self-regulate is disrupted when loneliness persists, which Cacioppo states can make us feel insecure and begin to scan for threats or dangers in our social landscape. He says that loneliness "causes us to apply these defensive perceptions to situations that are neutral or benign".[6] As a result, we become socially awk-ward, compounding the problem, as we inevitably push people away from us (yep, the *exact opposite* of what we want to happen). Perhaps we are wired to self-regulate so we can gain social acceptance.

Since arriving in Australia as a young immigrant boy from the Philippines, I faced a certain kind of discrimination and got picked on in high school for being 'different'. Some kids would pick on me for wearing glasses or tease me for my accent, while others would call me a 'nipper' to my face, which is a derogatory term used by kids back then for Asian people. Nipper came from the word Nippon which is a Japanese name for Japan. Of course, I wasn't even Japanese, but that never stopped those kids from saying it. Joining in Year 7 meant that most of the kids already knew each other, so I was the outsider. And since English wasn't my first language—Tagalog was always the spoken language at home—I found it even harder to fit in. As you can imagine, this caused considerable stress and anxiety for me grow-ing up. To avoid ridicule and keep out of the spotlight, which to me meant danger in the sense of psychological harm, I decided to stay quiet unless spoken to. And quiet I stayed until I was 25 years old (months after I moved to Sydney). Was I socially awkward for those 15 years? Yes, I was. But did I also long to have friends and belong to a group? Yes, I did. But for the sake of self-preservation, the vibrant boy who used to be more open and laughed and played with the other kids during his childhood became more withdrawn and antisocial, which then spiralled down into social disconnection.

Interestingly, in one of Cacioppo's loneliness studies, 'Loneliness within a nomological net: An evolutionary perspective'[7], 135 students undertook an array of psychological tests, with the results uncovering a broad spectrum of loneliness scores and traits. Digging deeper, the characteristics they found most likely to accompany loneliness included: depressed affect, shyness, low self-esteem, anxiety, hostility, pessimism, low agreeableness, introversion and fear of negative evaluation.[8] In addition, the study showed that students with higher loneliness scores also reported lower levels of social support, poorer social skills, higher anger, and higher negative mood compared to those low in loneliness.[9]

As I read through these findings, I began to tick off many of the unpleasant characteristics in my head from the time I went through loneliness. What particularly stood out for me was Cacioppo's positive correlation between loneliness and anger. I never quite understood how I became prone to this embarrassing behaviour, but I know it started to manifest in my late teens. I was a regular happy-go-lucky kid prior to coming to Australia but, somehow, it's as if I learned to become angry. My first memory of this intense feeling of anger was when I was driving not long after I'd gotten my driver's licence and was rudely cut off by another driver. I hate to admit it, but I was so enraged by his behaviour, that I started chasing him down several streets in my car. I must have been simmering inside like a pressure cooker that whole time and this situation finally triggered a blow-up. My emotions went haywire and any trace of self-regulation went out the door. It was like I'd had enough of the world taking advantage of me and I felt like this time I finally had the power to put an end to it. As I look back on it now, maybe the guy wasn't even trying to cut me off, or maybe he was—it doesn't really matter. As I learn more about the topic, I've discovered that loneliness can make us feel more vulnerable, behave more defensively and reduce our ability to think clearly. I realise now that all I really wanted was to be accepted. Perhaps after feeling on the outer for so long, my anger was a call for help, a call for friendships.

Have you ever watched footage of rescuers finding an abandoned or abused dog? At first, you see the animal behave defensively, growling and snarling or cowering to protect itself. Then as time passes and it realises the individual isn't a threat, its behaviour starts to change and it starts letting the person touch them. It begins to show more confidence, developing a trusting relationship with the carer over time, and (hopefully) it goes on to live happily ever after. In simplistic terms, I think we become a bit like this when we're lonely. At first, we scan for threats, we bite back from time to time to defend ourselves, but what we truly long for are deep connections that make us feel safe, loved and supported.

American Social Psychologist Roy Baumeister conducted a series of experiments with his colleagues on the effects of social rejection and exclusion on 259 psychology students with a median age of around 19 years. They manipulated social exclusion by telling the students that "they would either end up alone later in life or that other participants had rejected them".[10] In one experiment, some individuals were told: "I hate to tell you this, but no one chose you as someone they wanted to work with".[11] As you might guess, the impacts on their subjects' behaviours towards others were destructive: rejected people became more aggressive towards others, and were less likely to help or cooperate, whether it was the act of donating money or simply bending over to pick up pencils after the experimenter accidentally spilled a jar of them on the floor. Specifically, participants who were conditioned to think they were the type who would not have any friends in the future picked up less than one pencil each on average. Many just sat there and did nothing. Meanwhile, participants who were told to expect a future filled with accidents and injuries still got down on the floor and picked up eight or nine pencils on average.

So, what caused those who were told they would be alone later in life to *not* be willing to help someone out? Could their self-regulation (remember, our ability to control our thoughts and manage our emotions) be transiently disrupted at the thought of feeling rejected, thus throwing prosocial behaviours out the door? Well, the authors think the participants must have become wary and untrusting, as social exclusion may produce a temporary and protective absence of emotion, thus reducing their empathy and trust. Empathy allows us to understand the feelings of others. Without it, people can lose that desire to help. And without trust, these participants possibly became antisocial to reduce the risk of being hurt or being taken advantage of. This experiment makes me wonder: if loneliness and social exclusion make us more self-centred and less helpful towards others, what would the repercussions be, say in a relationship, in the workplace or in the broader community? What are the kinds of attitudes and behaviours we'd expect to see? I explore these ripple effects further in Chapter 7.

Roy's studies also showed that in addition to suppressing helpful behaviours, the experience or anticipation of social rejection also hampered intellectual performance. Participants exhibited large drops in logical reasoning, attention control, speed and accuracy, and poorer performance at controlled mental processes on tasks where the participant was required to regulate their thinking process. The results indicate that the thought of being alone can undermine our ability to think clearly. This could help to explain why I started failing university subjects after my relationship breakup. I remember just how difficult it became to concentrate on my studies. I would read a book, and yet I was unable to process any of the information, even if I read the same content repeatedly. It might have even contributed to my second car accident, where I completely misjudged the speed of the oncoming car.

ON THE BODY

Our body also suffers when our need for connection is unmet. When we are unable to self-regulate, Cacioppo says we become vulnerable to stressors which "act as a corrosive force that accelerates the aging process".[12] Right down to the very molecular level of ourselves, this inability to self-regulate disrupts key cellular processes in our bodies, predisposing us to premature aging. But what exactly is going on, which makes us age so quickly during chronic loneliness?

In one of Cacioppo's experiments, he recruited and observed lonely and non-lonely young adults in a sleep lab. The study revealed that lonely people took longer to fall asleep, accompanied by feelings of greater daytime fatigue.[13] Interestingly, even though the quantity of sleep was the same across both groups, the lonely group had lower *quality* of sleep, thus they didn't feel refreshed from their slumber (a feeling I recollect all too well). Extending Cacioppo's link between loneliness, lack of sleep and accelerated ageing, a study done by researchers at UCLA in 29 adults aged between 61 and 86 discovered that even just a single night of insufficient sleep made the subjects' cells age more quickly.[14]

It doesn't stop there. A study conducted by Social Epidemiologist Lisa Berkman found that people who lacked social and community ties were *more likely to die* in a nine-year follow-up period, independent of people's socioeconomic or physical health status.[15] More specifically, according to Cacioppo, people with fewer social ties have an increased risk of dying from ischemic heart disease, cerebrovascular and circulatory disease, cancer, and gastrointestinal and respiratory issues.[16]

So, what's the link between loneliness and these downstream effects on our health?

It appears that the chronic stress caused by perceived loneliness plays a key role. In one study, Capiocco's team found higher traces of the stress hormone adrenaline in the morning urine of older adults experiencing perceived loneliness.[17]

Research has also linked loneliness and social isolation to a weakened immune system. In a 2005 study of 83 first-semester healthy university students, those with both high levels of loneliness and a small social network had the lowest antibody response to an influenza vaccine.[18] Being socially connected is not only good for your emotional wellbeing but it also has a significant influence on your physical body. Psychology Professor Julianne Holt-Lunstad, one of the world's leading researchers on social connection, summed it up well: "Just like being physically active, we need to be socially active".[19]

Feeling lonely also affects the body's cardiovascular system. Not only is it bad for your figurative heart, but your literal one as well.

Cacioppo explains that loneliness penetrates our cells by making changes in our DNA transcription, which then makes changes to the cells' sensitivity to cortisol, dampening the ability to shut off the body's inflammatory response.[20] And, when inflammation becomes chronic it promotes cardiovascular disease.

Cacioppo also discovered that loneliness doesn't just damage the cardiovascular system through stress, but also when an individual tries to cope passively with that stress (i.e. enduring it without trying to change their situation). People who feel lonely are more likely to cope passively, and this has its consequences. Specifically, their blood pressure rises by constricting the small blood vessels throughout the body (otherwise known as increasing total peripheral resistance), which in turn forces the heart to work harder to pump blood through that constricted circulatory system.[21] In Cacioppo's studies with Ohio State University students, those with higher levels of loneliness were found to also have higher total peripheral resistance. So, while acute stress can be a good thing to keep us alert and motivated to perform day-to-day tasks, chronic stress as a result of long-term loneliness, combined with passive coping, can actually shorten our lifespan due to the wear and tear it places on our bodies. Chronic loneliness is *a silent killer*.

When Psychologist Martha McClintock and her colleagues at the University of Chicago studied female Sprague-Dawley rats living alone or in groups, they discovered breast tumours in the socially isolated rats, which were 84 times larger than those of rats housed together, as measured by weight. The study also revealed an increase of 135 percent in the number of discrete tumour masses in socially isolated rats.[22] This example highlights what experiences of isolation can make us susceptible to and what it has the potential to do to our bodies if we don't socially reconnect. It appears, too, that the link between isolation and cancer risk is strong in women, but not necessarily men.[23, 24] That is, women who are socially isolated have an increased risk of dying from cancer. Though men's cancer incidence isn't necessarily linked with social isolation, unsurprisingly, those with fewer connections appear to have poorer cancer survival rates.

I saw these statistics play out in my own family. In 2008, my mother, Cora, was diagnosed with breast cancer and, although there were other factors at play, given the evidence, I can't shrug off the impact social isolation must have had on her health. Removed from the only world she'd ever known, and without a job or the company of her old friends and family in Manila, Mum fell into a severe depression for a very long time (I will explain more of her story in Chapter 7). My mother's breast cancer diagnosis was one of the scariest pieces of news I've had the displeasure of receiving. When I was a young boy, I used to believe that my parents were invincible—they were my superheroes. So, when Dad called to say that Mum had breast cancer, I was devastated. I'd already been living in Sydney for a few years at the time; the global financial crisis had just begun, and I lost my job in the process. After dealing from the various traumas I had been through in Melbourne, it felt like one of the worst and most stressful years of my life. To make matters worse, Mum isolated herself even further from family and friends. For whatever reason, she didn't want anyone to know what she was going through, not even her own brothers and sisters.

During the chemo stages, Mum completely retreated at home, mostly staying in the bedroom where she could hide herself away from everyone. It was a complete blow to the family. What was going through her head at the time I can only speculate, but what I know for sure was that she wasn't in the right frame of mind. Relatives and friends would ring but she wouldn't answer the phone. They would come for a visit but she refused to come downstairs and greet them, so Dad would have to make up an excuse that Mum was sleeping. This continued for months and people were getting worried.

I recall visiting my parents in Melbourne to see how Mum was going, and it wasn't good. She'd not only lost weight and her hair—which was bad enough in itself—but her behaviour had totally changed. She was extremely irritable and inconsolable—at times she would get so angry, screaming at Dad in order to complain about the littlest things. Her behaviour got so bad it reduced him to tears. I realised at that point that Dad needed my support as well. Sometimes we only think about caring for those going through cancer but we forget to think about how much their carers need our support too, for their own wellbeing. As my brothers and I had moved out of home already, and with Mum isolating herself from family and friends, Dad was left with the difficult task of looking after her needs all by himself. With what I saw of my mum in just a few days, I can only imagine what Dad would have had to shoulder alone on a daily basis.

At a time when she could have benefited from being in the company of others, not only did Mum isolate herself, but she dragged Dad down that same lonely path as well. I flew back to Sydney thinking about how I should consider moving back to Melbourne, so I could be closer to my parents and be there to support them.

A few months later, my phone rang, and Dad was on the other line. My heart pounded. "Is Mum okay?" I wondered anxiously.

"Joel, I just called to say that your mama is healed. Her chemo worked and she no longer has cancer," he said.

I was so relieved. Not only was I happy for Mum, but I was relieved it was over for Dad's sake and for his mental health, too. I am glad to report that it's been ten-plus years since then and Mum is still cancer-free! Like a phoenix risen from the ashes, she's back—physically and mentally—now rocking healthy long white hair and a completely new outlook on life. As if the scales have been removed from her eyes, she's a completely changed woman now, a much happier person like how I remembered her to be when I was a young boy.

I can't help but think that perhaps the social disconnection and isolation she felt here in Australia contributed to her getting breast cancer, but I can only speculate. As the evidence in both animals and humans has shown us, this kind of social environmental change truly can have an influence on the development of tumours. But being sociable doesn't necessarily protect us entirely against cancer, although it does make me think of just how important relationships are to our survival. How much more evidence do we need?

In one particular study in 2010 called 'Social Relationships and Mortality Risk: A Meta-analytic Review'[25], researchers tracked the social habits of more than 300,000 people worldwide over a seven-and-a-half-year period. What they found was that individuals with stronger social relationships showed a 50 percent increased likelihood of surviving compared to those with poor or insufficient relationships. In other words, the quality of one's social relationships is not only good for our mental health but it's also linked to our mortality. I'm thankful Mum survived; but, as this study indicates, isolating yourself isn't a risk worth taking.

THE BLUE ZONE

Across our planet are five discrete regions that share a unique bond: their populations consist of a higher-than-average number of centenarians.

Cente-what? you ask. Essentially, it's people who live over the age of 100.

These regions were dubbed 'Blue Zones' by National Geographic Explorer Dan Buettner after he and his colleagues discovered and drew blue circles around hotspots of villages across the world whose citizens demonstrated the highest longevity. One of those blue zones, where the highest concentration of men live equally as long as the women past the age of 100, lies in the mountainous villages of the Italian island of Sardinia, in the Mediterranean Sea.

Browsing through TEDx videos on loneliness and social wellbeing, I came across Susan Pinker, psychologist and author of 'The Village Effect'.[26] In her talk, she discusses these particular villages in Sardinia, which have captivated the world over due to their high concentrations of healthy centenarians, specifically men, given elsewhere in the world men are outlived by their wives and sisters by up to 20 or 30 years. Although earlier research suggested that the inhabitants' longevity was in part due to their Mediterranean diet (fruits, vegetables, whole grains, beans, nuts, and legumes),

Susan's curiosity was piqued, so she decided to research the whole lifestyle of Sardinians, quickly discovering another critical factor to their long, healthy lives. When she visited their villages, one of the first things she noticed was the densely and tightly spaced houses where people's lives constantly intersected. Susan found that, rather than it being a matter of simply thinking positively that kept Sardinians alive and healthier for longer, it was their social connectedness that underpinned their longevity. Across their lifespan and as people aged, they were constantly integrated within the community, surrounded by family, friends, neighbours and many others. Summed up succinctly: "*They are never left to live solitary lives*". What a stark contrast to our culture in Australia, where ageing is not celebrated and the elderly are faced with increasing social exclusion. Growing up in the Philippines, people are brought up to respect and look after their elderly—less out of duty, and more out of love. In Australia, however, our elderly parents either live on their own or are checked into nursing homes, which only aggravates the loneliness situation as they're further isolated in the process. In places like Sardinia, surrounding the elderly with family, friends and neighbours not only helps to curb loneliness but prolongs their lives, as Susan pointed out.

While I don't have the silver bullet as to how we can replicate Sardinia's lifestyle here in Australia long-term—as sadly it's just how our society and culture operate at the moment—I will share some strategies in a later chapter of the book about how we can alleviate chronic loneliness in our society.

ON THE BRAIN

Not only does loneliness affect our bodies and behaviours, but also the physical health signalling pathways and structures of our brain. A study conducted by Angelina Sutin, associate professor at the College of Medicine at Florida State University, showed that feeling lonely is associated with increasing your risk of dementia by 40 percent.[27] The study involved data from 12,000 participants (Americans 50 years and older and their spouses) collected over a ten-year period. During that time 1,104 people developed dementia, a condition characterised by a decline in memory, language and other thinking skills. Participants who recorded subjective feelings of isolation had an increased risk of developing dementia. This was distinct from the degree of social connectedness or number of contacts and goes to show how important *deep and meaningful* social relationships are in keeping our minds engaged in a way that promotes and maintains cognitive health and function. As the saying goes: 'use it or lose it'.

Curious to see whether science has yet unearthed how 'feeling lonely' looks in the brain's signalling patterns, I came across two functional MRI studies fortuitously published during the COVID-19 pandemic.

The first, out of Dartmouth Social Neuroscience Laboratory[28], looked at how loneliness affects people's 'neural map' or perception of themselves versus others and discovered that when we're socially integrated, the region of our medial prefrontal brain that lights up when we think of our individual self shows a high similarity to when we think of the people closest to us—there's *literally* a strong connection between us and our loved ones. For participants of the study who were feeling lonelier, their brain maps showed reduced overlap between the area which lit up when thinking of themselves versus their loved ones, giving a whole new meaning to the sense of disconnectedness lonely people say they feel, even when surrounded by others. I'm not surprised to see these findings when I think back on my own experiences and feelings of disconnection from family and friends, and when I hear from others in my network who've reflected similar sentiments. It is strangely reassuring though, to have a glimpse of what's going on behind the scenes, in our minds.

The second study, published in Nature later in 2020, examined the similarities in brain regions activated by deprivation of food and social contact.[29] It turns out, just as Michelle had suggested, that when we are forced to be isolated, we crave social interactions in much the same way a hungry person craves food. Participants' midbrain dopaminergic regions, called the substantia nigra and ventral tegmental areas, were lit up like Christmas trees during their functional MRI scans after they were deprived of food or social interaction (face-to-face and digital) for ten hours. This means that acute, forced loneliness activates some kind of 'craving circuit'. Interestingly, and somewhat sadly, individuals who reported higher levels of pre-existing chronic loneliness demonstrated more subdued midbrain responses in the study, although it's still unclear whether their loneliness caused the low responsiveness to social cues, or if they were already wired in such a way that predisposed them to loneliness. Maybe there are cases of both in our world—either way, I have a real and living hope that chronic loneliness is a circuit we can most certainly break.

My aim in this chapter was to highlight how loneliness isn't just a temporary situation or problem people have from time to time, but a serious and tangible issue that demands our attention. I have shared but a portion of all the research available in the world on loneliness. The more I read, the more I see how significant this topic is. The more I understand, the more I must do something about it. Chronic loneliness is a disease that needs a cure. My hope is that by now you have seen and heard enough to realise its devastating effects on the mind and body. Not only does it affect the individual, but its ripples extend to touch those around and beyond them. ♣

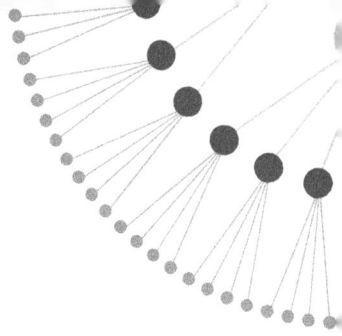

CHAPTER 5

Why Do We Get Lonely?

IT'S IN OUR DNA

We know by now that humans are social beings, but to answer the question of how deeply embedded our need for social connection is, we must first travel way back in time to when our species began to roam the earth.

According to the theory of evolution, Homo sapiens evolved from ape-like ancestors, but eventually outlived all other species of the human race, including Neanderthals who died out approximately 30,000 years ago. Though there is still debate around how they died off, archaeological evidence shows Neanderthals shared something in common with us, which allowed them to stay safe, resilient and survive for over 300,000 years: they lived together in groups[1]. Sadly, their numbers dwindled to a point of no return and they became history. Meanwhile, modern humans eventually learned to cooperate and develop language, coming up with innovative solutions to problems in order to better adapt to our environment and survive. For example, our creation of the humble bone needle allowed us to sew and tailor animal skins together to keep the heat in. As we worked together, we were able to create more sophisticated weapons for hunting animals big and small, which were crucial to our survival in the last Ice Age.

I can't imagine what life must have been like during that period for humans, a time when glaciers covered huge parts of the planet. With all our creature comforts today, I'll never complain about winter again! Not only did our ancestors have to thrive in cold, harsh climates but they also had to compete with other predators—including sabre tooth tigers, lions, bears and wolves—to stay alive. Despite these unimaginable conditions, our species survived. In fact, we flourished, especially after the last Ice Age period ended about 11,000 to 12,000 years ago[2], and more favourable conditions allowed us to evolve from hunter-gatherers to farmers cultivating crops. This lifestyle shift resulted in our ancestors building more permanent dwellings, communities and societies. It was also a catalyst for us to learn to cooperate and build relationships with people outside our immediate clans and families, extending our circles to other groups from near and far who also dwelt in these settled societies.

Now, if we add up all those tens of thousands of years our species spent time together for survival, it becomes easier to understand how our need for social connection has been

handed down and reinforced from generation to generation. But as I found out, it goes even deeper than that—
to the molecular level. So much so that Cacioppo says, "The
genetic propensity for desiring social connection and the
propensity for feeling social pain in its absence are transmit-
ted through bits of genetic information in our cells, coded
as instructions for making proteins".[3] In other words, our
desire for connection is *hardwired* in us, which is why we
feel lonely when we get separated from the pack.

Fast-forward to the last two centuries, when industri-
alisation accelerated the migration of people to work in
cities. I see it the most in my own people, moving far away
from the family home to countries on the other side of the
world just for that 'right' opportunity to earn a living—as
if the right job can't exist anywhere else. In the process, we
become lonely as we get physically disconnected from the
towns, villages and people we hold so dear. We may have
dramatically changed our environment over the last few
centuries, and our technology may have advanced in leaps
and bounds, but underneath our organic cotton shirts and
RM Williams boots, our physiology remains the same.

This is why Cacioppo said disconnection leads to such
dysregulation and damage, down to the cellular level. He
explained how this gene expression is dependent on environmental factors, otherwise known as epigenetics. For
example, the proteins that carry messages in our blood and
our nervous system take on the form of hormones and neurotransmitters such as adrenaline, oxytocin and serotonin,
all of which serve a purpose in guiding and prompting

specific behavioural responses in us, such as bonding in larger groups, or looking after our human offspring so that our children may survive. So, when we experience the disconnectedness of moving cities for work or relying solely on technology to sustain our relationships, these experiences interact with our genes to produce protein messages that manifest in behaviours to alleviate the loneliness.

Bringing this back to the early Homo sapiens, to manage our world's increasingly complex social structures, our growing 'social brain'—visible as an expanded cerebral cortex—gave us the advantage of learning by social observation, recognising the shifting status of friends and foes, orchestrating relationships, adhering to social norms, and sacrificing one's self-interest for the interest of a partner or social group, in exchange for the possibility of long term mutual benefits.[4] Interestingly, the frontal brain areas relied upon for these social skills are most impeded during experiences of social isolation.

So, although being social is 'in our DNA', and not just a practice passed from generation to generation, it is important to note that genes are unlikely to have a direct effect on loneliness in and of themselves. Rather, it's how they are expressed in response to our social environments, such as the homes we grow up in or the circles and communities we dwell in. Yet even in the light of this complex, dynamic and interactive sense of our genetics, we can still say we truly are social creatures by design.

AT A GLOBAL SCALE

Okay, so we've determined that our desire for connection involves our genes, the very blueprint of our being. This means loneliness isn't an issue exclusive to people in Australia, but a common experience that binds us across the planet.

Here's a snapshot of global statistics to prove it:

In the US, a survey of more than 20,000 adults revealed that nearly half of respondents sometimes or always felt alone or left out.[5] In England, 45 percent of adults feel occasionally, sometimes or often lonely. That's about twenty-five million people.[6] Due to the burden of the region's ever-increasing loneliness, the UK even appointed the world's first Minister for Loneliness in 2018.

Across Europe, the European Commission found that 7 percent or approximately thirty million adults frequently feel lonely.[7] In their report, loneliness was found to be more prevalent in Eastern (Bulgaria, Czech Republic, Croatia, Estonia, Hungary, Lithuania, Poland, Slovenia and Slovakia) and Southern Europe (Cyprus, Greece, Italy, Portugal and Spain) than Western (Austria, Germany, France, Belgium and the Netherlands) and Northern Europe (Denmark, Finland, Ireland, Sweden and the UK). A combination of poorer health, economic conditions and living alone were associated with higher rates of loneliness, suggesting it's not just a problem for developed nations.

Closer to home, Japan, too, struggles with loneliness. Statistics focusing on this problem are scarce in Japan;

however, an estimated 18.4 million adults currently live alone.[8, 9] The consequence of this solo dwelling has tragically given rise to 'kodokushi'—a Japanese term used to describe when people die alone, undiscovered for long periods of time. It breaks my heart that a word such as this even exists.

Finally, our closest neighbour, New Zealand, shared in their Ministry of Social Development's Social Report that 13.9 percent of their population aged 15 years and over have felt lonely all, most or some of the time during the last four weeks.[10]

Interestingly, I was not able to find loneliness statistics or published research for many countries, and it wasn't for lack of trying. It suggests to me that most parts of the world are yet to put more emphasis on the subject or are only just beginning to take loneliness seriously as a major contributor to mental health decline.

The available evidence also shows that loneliness affects *all* age groups across the planet, which makes sense, as we found earlier, given our need for social connections is built into our DNA and is constantly interacting with our environment throughout our entire lifespan. In the early stages of writing *Better Together*, many people were quick to share with me how they associated loneliness with old age. On the contrary, wherever research has been conducted across age groups, findings have shown time and again that *younger* people appear to experience the highest levels of loneliness. Surprised? Don't be—I'll talk you through the reasons why in the next chapter.

Not meaning to get off-topic, but is it a coincidence that with all this loneliness going on in the world that depression too is at an all-time high? I think not. The World Health Organisation states that depression is now the leading cause of disability worldwide with more than three hundred million people of all ages globally suffering from depression.[11] In a research study entitled 'Perceived social isolation, evolutionary fitness and health outcomes: a lifespan approach', Psychologist Louise Hawkley pointed to evidence linking perceived loneliness with adverse health effects including depression (as well as cognitive decline, poor sleep quality, poor cardiovascular function and impaired immunity at every stage of life) as it wreaks havoc on an individual's physical, mental and cognitive health.[12]

When speaking with Dr Zoya Jamshidi, a clinical and counselling psychologist who runs a practice in Sydney's North Shore, I asked her, "In your ten years' experience dealing with patients (young and old), what do you think is the common theme in their situations? Why do they come to you?"

Zoya replied with a single word: "Relationships," which was followed by a pause, then, "or lack thereof".

I was stunned—in the silence that followed, you could hear a pin drop. It wasn't the response I'd expected, but it was the one I needed to crystalise the common thread that was woven throughout my findings for the book. The conversation I had that day confirmed for me that if we *ever* want to stand a chance in decreasing the levels of loneliness and depression in our world, then we *must* make social wellbeing a priority and start to think about ways we can help build meaningful relationships in our lives. Our survival depends on it. Sadly though, so many people in society don't even have a confidant to talk to, someone who 'feels like home'.

It's such a blessing we have specialists like Dr Jamshidi who we can reach out to for help and counselling. But doctors and psychologists are not 'friends': they have a professional relationship with us to help us understand and deal with our problems—really, a *one-way* relationship. According to Relationship Australia, a good relationship includes companionship and mutual emotional support.[13] This is a *two-way* relationship that goes beyond professional services, and the kind we need to find and nurture outside of the doctor's office if we are to lead longer, healthier and happier lives.

THE DIGITAL WORLD

In a world where we are increasingly living alone and working from home, could digital tools help us to stay better connected and nurture deep and meaningful two-way relationships?

Many people think not. This is much talked about in the book *Alone Together*, written by Sherry Turkle, who is a professor of social studies of science and technology at MIT. The book's oxymoronic title refers to technology as something that promises to bring us closer yet leaves many of us feeling less connected. Consider social media app Facebook, whose mission is to: "Give people the power to build community and bring the world closer together".[14] On one hand, the platform is meant to make it easier for us to engage with thousands of others but, on the other, it also makes it easier to avoid face-to-face contact.

It's happening with smartphones too. Instead of calling people, we often prefer to text them instead. According to Professor Turkle, at a screen, we feel protected and less burdened by expectations. Elaine, 17, one of Professor Turkle's interviewees, said that the screen "is a place to hide".[15] Elaine explains, "When you can think about what you're going to say, you can talk [write] to someone you'd have trouble talking to".

Elaine is right in that the advantage of communicating using text means we can reflect, retype and edit before sending, and the other person never needs to know the number of times the message was revised. It reminds me of Microsoft Teams, the collaboration and communication tool we use at work. Many times I have fallen into the same habit of messaging my colleagues on the program instead of walking up to them to talk—even though they are only *a few feet* away! We are beginning to rely so much on instant messaging that we risk losing the all-important face-to-face contact that builds rapport and helps form lasting bonds. And the more technology becomes intertwined in our daily lives, the more we become overstimulated by and tethered to it.

One of Professor Turkle's interviewees, Roman, 18, said, "If I get a Facebook message or something posted on my wall, I have to see it. I have to". Roman then goes on to share that many of his classmates admit that they too are so glued to their phones that they get into accidents when walking. Does that ring a bell? It does for me. For many years, every time my phone buzzed, I had to look to see what it was all about. I needed to know who tried to contact me. I would scroll through my Facebook feed in fear of missing out, at times even zombie-scrolling just to fill up the minutes. The turning point for me was when my wife gave birth to our son, and I decided that no call, no text, no social media or work message was worth risking the safety of my family, especially when driving. So, for the past three years, I have been stowing my phone inside the car's centre console—out of sight and out of mind.

Sometimes I wish we were back in the simpler times of the eighties. When I was growing up, I couldn't wait to run outside to play with friends, ride bicycles, play with marbles or matchbox cars, or play hide and seek with the other kids in the neighbourhood. We learned to use our imaginations for entertainment to combat boredom and make our own fun. Fast forward to today and we're struggling to get kids to go outside anymore. Technology is increasingly keeping all of us indoors, tethered to whatever is consuming us on our devices.

Isn't it scary to think of how *everything* is on a tiny mobile device, which we so badly depend on? Games, movies, music, social interactions, our work apps and data … some people even say that they only need their phone to run their business these days. No wonder we're so obsessed with our devices that we get anxious when we don't have them in our pockets, or we panic when we think we've lost them. As we choose to be glued more frequently to our screens indoors and for longer periods, the fewer people we meet within the real world. Our ancestors would turn in their graves to learn how disconnected we are becoming.

Can you imagine what it would be like if the last ten years of our existence were showcased inside a museum? Picture an exhibit of a family: in one display, a teenage girl is scrolling through endless images on Instagram in her bedroom; in the next room, her brother is watching Netflix on his laptop while eating dinner in bed; in the kitchen, their mother eats supper on her own as their father sits on the couch answering emails—'luckily' she has Facebook to scroll through and keep her company.

In another part of the museum, we see a display of our ancestors: they are eating supper together as a family inside their wooden hut with a thatched roof; in another display, kids are playing merrily out in the open while their parents and other tribe members are gathered around a campfire, talking, laughing and singing into the moonlight.

Can you visualise the stark contrast of interactions between our ancestors and us today? Which group would you rather be part of? Where would you feel a stronger sense of belonging?

Our advances in digital technology allowed us to progress in leaps and bounds and even landed us on the moon, but while we made this giant leap for mankind, the same powerful tool is pulling our relationships apart ... and yet, we wonder why loneliness is becoming an epidemic.

If we truly want to improve the state of wellbeing in our society, then what we need is a transformation around *how* we tackle the issue of mental health. We solve it not by throwing money at the same solutions over and over again, but by taking more of a holistic approach and including social wellbeing in our programs, surrounding ourselves with the right people, and creating a framework around awareness and education that will get us to a place where people can have deep and meaningful relationships with one another. As we explored at the beginning of this chapter, no matter how technologically advanced we become as a species, our biological desire for social connection and face-to-face contact does not change. It's inbuilt in us as a survival mechanism. ✤

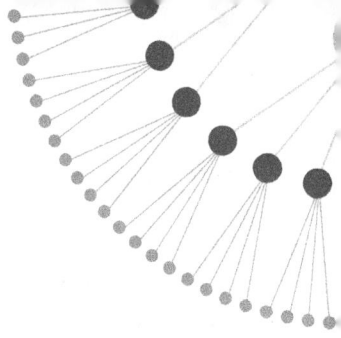

CHAPTER 6

Who is Vulnerable to Loneliness?

This chapter highlights the different life stages and groups of people that may be more vulnerable to loneliness. As we've come to realise, loneliness can affect anyone—the young and old alike. By providing you a glimpse into the kinds of situations that can lead us into experiencing elements of loneliness, my aim is to help you become more aware, understanding and empathetic when it occurs (whether to others or yourself) and, in the process, be part of the solution together.

Note: although a number of people groups are not specifically cited in this chapter, when we dig beneath the surface of it, many of the fundamental elements of loneliness are a shared experience across demographics and will resonate regardless of race, gender, age or region.

INFANTS AND CHILDREN

Just as our desire for human connection is demonstrated and passed down from generation to generation, we also see this need in children from a very young age, in fact right from the moment they are born. I witnessed this firsthand after the birth of our son, Logan.

Taken from the warmth and safety of his mother's womb, Logan began to cry within seconds of entering the world, feeling vulnerable and unprotected. But, as soon as he was reunited with Belinda and placed in her warm embrace, Logan miraculously began to calm down and breathe more slowly again. The nurse explained to us that this skin-to-skin contact had many positive benefits such as helping Logan to breastfeed more effectively and stabilising his skin temperature, heart rate and breathing rate in the process. Skin-to-skin contact also causes a release in oxytocin (the 'love hormone') when we snuggle up and gives a calming and bonding effect, thus countering the effects of cortisol (the 'stress hormone'), which soothes the baby, helping them to stop crying. Pretty cool to know, right?

As months went on, I noticed how Logan began to show signs of separation anxiety. This wasn't so much about loneliness—which children at that age don't fully comprehend yet—but rather the early indicators of our innate need to be in the company of others. From about six months of age, Logan would suddenly cry if he saw me move as little as three feet away from him and would only stop once I picked him up. I now understand what parents mean when they say kids want to be around you: *All. The. Time.* Like your shadow, so much so that you can't even spend a minute in private to yourself. One time, I slipped away quietly to use the bathroom, while Logan played with toys in the living room. Next thing, he came banging on the door, wedging his tiny little fingers through the cracks at the bottom saying, "Da-da … Da-DA!" I couldn't even be upset about it; it was so funny that I had to laugh. I had recollections of a scene from the movie *Sister Act* when Whoopi and the choir of nuns sang "I will follow him, follow him wherever he may go …". There was no escape, but I try to cherish moments like those because the time will come when he'll want to be independent and I'll be the one to chase him down for attention. Such is life.

Separation anxiety can affect parents too. I remember the first time Belinda and I left Logan with a nanny during a holiday in Fiji so we could spend some much-needed time together. Every fibre in me told me we shouldn't leave him; that Logan was vulnerable and couldn't fend for himself; that we didn't even know who this nanny was who we had entrusted our son with. What if she hurt him? How would we know? *What if she took him away and we never saw him again?*

I get it: every veteran parent who's ever had the privilege of visiting Fiji *knows* Fijians are the most loving, caring and gentle people when it comes to kids. They absolutely treasure them, and they absolutely treasured Logan. But anxious thoughts were running through my mind. Belinda was fending off her welling emotions with a healthy dose of pragmatism, while I put on a brave face and tried to be strong for the both of us. And, despite our anxieties, Logan survived the hour it took for our couples' massage *just fine* and relished in the attention his nanny and the other staff gave him.

The same thing happened again when we dropped him off on his first day at family care. Logan wailed as we walked away. It was heartbreaking seeing him that way. I imagined how scared he would have felt, wanting to say, "Mum, Dad, don't leave me! I don't know this woman. Come back!" but he couldn't. The only thing he could do was cry. Little did we know at the time, he stopped crying within minutes of us leaving. Perhaps it was indeed harder for us to leave him there than it was for him to stay.

Isn't it a shame that infants know how to cry for help when they want our company, yet somehow, we've grown to stop doing the same, not seeking support when we need it the most? We hide our tears and pains on the inside where they build up and wreak havoc on our mental health.

Logan is three years old now and has a little sister, Ruby. As difficult as it can be to raise children with all their melt-downs and the sleep-deprived nights, I realise now how good they can also be for our own mental and social wellbe-ing. My worldly problems and stresses melt away every time I come home—especially when I see Logan run towards me, smiling and giggling as he stretches his hands out wide for a cuddle with his sister toddling not far behind. It's the best feeling anyone could ever ask for. Where previously I stayed back late in the office, I now can't wait to be home on time so I can be with my family to have a bit of play, dinner, and read the kids bedtime stories before they go to sleep.

As it turns out, research shows that a child's improved vocabulary, reading and writing skills, as well as academic performance are linked to sitting down to family dinners, according to Susan Pinker, in her book *The Village Effect*.[1] Having healthy banter and discussion with your child during dinner boosts their literacy and language skills when compared to children whose parents' communication style is mostly to give orders at the dinner table: sit, eat your food, chew with your mouth closed, end of conversation.

There are other benefits too. In one study, Guang Guo, an American sociologist, examined the link between a certain set of genes and delinquent, violent behaviour in adolescent boys in the US, as well as the influence of subjects' home and social environments on their genetic propensities.[2] His team studied 1,100 boys in Grades 7 to 12, and found specific variations in three dopamine system genes that were associated with delinquent and violent behaviour, but only when subjects suffered some form of stress, such as ongoing family issues, low popularity or failing school. Specifically, Guo and his team learned that a certain mutation in one of the genes was most influential when a boy did not have regular meals with his family. In an interview with Reuters, Guo explained, "But if people with the same gene have a parent who has regular meals with them, then the risk [of delinquent, violent behaviour] is gone".[3] It's fascinating to see how strongly our home life moderates our gene expression, but I'm also not so surprised by this finding. Genes should never be an excuse for bad behaviour, but rather highlight the importance of having nurturing parents in our children's lives. Too often I hear people judge kids for their actions, but I argue that we need to be educating parents more on how to raise children with a deep sense of home, belonging, boundaries and accountability. The problem we face is that parents often aren't willing or able to seek outside help and invest the necessary time and effort to change habits and lifestyle.

An even greater problem exists when children don't have parents or role models by their side to begin with. In a study supporting the practice of regular family mealtimes, American Psychologist and Eating Disorder Expert Debra Franko followed close to 2,400 girls from ages nine to nineteen and found that frequent family meals in the first three years of the study played a factor in the child's personal development in years to come. In particular, the girls who said they "never or almost never ate" with their parents between the ages of nine and eleven were more likely to become teenagers who were stressed-out, smokers, or demonstrated disordered attitudes toward food.[4]

These findings (and many, many more)[5] go to show *just how important family dinners are* in helping our children not only become good citizens or academically successful but to be psychologically healthier as well. Mealtimes give parents the chance to be role models, reinforce positive values and provide a support system to each family member.

One particular woman whose products have become a household name, thanks her father for these dinner table conversations. When Sara was growing up, her dad would encourage her to fail. I know, it sounds kind of bad—but let me explain why. Sara would come home from school each day, sit at the dinner table and her father would ask her and her brother what they failed at that day. If they didn't have something to tell him, he'd express his disappointment. What she didn't realise at the time was that her dad was redefining what failure meant for them—that if they weren't failing enough, they weren't trying new things—and she came to realise that the only failure was if she didn't try at all. Emboldened by her upbringing, Sara went on to try many things in life unafraid, knowing that even if she failed, her dad would be okay with it, praising her efforts and proud of her no matter what.

That woman is none other than Sara Blakely, the world's youngest self-made billionaire, who founded the hugely successful shapewear company, Spanx. Now, I'm not saying we should have family dinners just so our kids can go on to become billionaires, but who would have thought that her success began at the family dinner table?

YOUNG PEOPLE

As we learned in Chapter 6, perhaps surprisingly, research shows young people have the highest levels of experiencing loneliness. For the purpose of this chapter, I'm loosely referring to youth aged 12 to 24 years old (i.e. high school to university age). At this time of their lives, their brains are still developing and they may not yet be as resilient to challenges as older adults.

When I interviewed Dr Michelle Lim, I asked the all-important question: how many quality relationships does one need to have to be happy? And, of course, the answer was that *it depends*: "Well, young people focus on having many friends but with less quality, while older people prefer fewer, but seek deeper relationships".

So, with a need for many friends and to be accepted by peers, on top of academic pressures, body changes, family situations and environmental factors, it's no wonder that so many young people are at risk of psychological distress and worse, suicide—the leading cause of death in young Australians.[6]

JAKE'S STORY

Let me share with you a conversation I had with a friend of mine who went through depression as a teenager. To protect his identity, we'll call him Jake. Jake and I met and developed a friendship through our mutual passion for motorcycles.

Born in Australia to Kiwi parents, Jake and his family moved to Singapore during his teenage years, while his father worked there as an expat. When Jake was 16, his family had a big family lunch on Christmas Day. During the lunch, the conversation turned sour. Jake learned about some horrible things that had happened to his family in the past caused by his uncle, which ended in a huge fight between his uncle and his parents, and left relationships in his family completely severed. His uncle walked out and

Jake never heard from him again. What hurt the most for Jake was that his uncle was an important figure to him, and to lose his uncle in his life so suddenly through no fault of his own was a traumatic experience.

In the following year, Jake met his first girlfriend in Singapore, but within months she ended up cheating on him. "I was the last person in school to find out." In the process, Jake lost some friends who were also friends with his ex-girlfriend. "So, a mixture of these events, along with the increasingly tense environment at school as I was in my final year ... I cracked. I cracked hard. It was actually before we even broke up, I began to feel depressed. It was a few months of feeling extremely low before I was able to say, 'Yeah, I think this is worse than just being sad'."

In just a short period of time, Jake got the triple whammy of breakdowns: not only in family relationships, but with a girlfriend, and his friendships too. On top of that, he was living abroad, which was already pretty isolating and untethering in itself. Jake was devastated and felt completely alone. His family noticed he was not his usual self and took him straight to a psychiatrist, who prescribed him antidepressants after Jake explained he was having suicidal thoughts.

"There were a few occasions where I wanted to die, but one night in particular I thought, 'Yep, I'm going to do it'. My parents instantly figured out what was happening, called my psychiatrist and got me booked in a mental hospital at the Institute of Mental Health in Singapore," Jake explained.

"I will never forget my experience there, but one of the worst memories was when Dad drove me there. He was so angry. He didn't know how to react to this. I could only tell him that he didn't understand how bad I really felt."

My heart broke for Jake when he shared about the car ride to the hospital. His dad told him that he was acting up and that he felt embarrassed for the way Jake was behaving. I wonder how many parents out there react the same way as his father did. Jake said this made it even harder for him to open up to his dad afterwards.

Jake spent a few weeks at the hospital where he saw some very ill patients in even worse conditions than him, which really helped to put things in perspective. "It wouldn't be weird for someone to have a schizophrenic episode or for someone to find a way to cut themselves a few meters away from me. After three weeks, I woke up one morning, feeling just a bit better, enough for me to want to go outside, to walk, to talk to my family. The next day I was able to leave the Institute."

What he shared next sent chills down my spine as it brought back unpleasant memories of something I had also experienced: "Unfortunately, my depression continued on, even becoming worse for a while where I began to experience hearing voices and seeing things such as people. But I didn't want to die—I was just living with it".

Can you imagine what that would have been like for him? Maybe like a scene from *The Sixth Sense* where the young boy, Cole, was seeing the dead nobody else could. His most memorable line in the movie was to his psychiatrist, Malcolm: "I wanna tell you my secret now ... I see dead people".

As I shared in Chapter 5, I began seeing things whilst suffering from chronic loneliness and depression. Hearing Jake share his similar experience felt close to home. Until that point, I had thought I was the only one in my network of friends and family who had ever experienced such hallucinations. If Jake's psychiatrist determined that he was schizophrenic at the time, then it makes me wonder what I could have had, even transiently. I'll never know for sure as I never sought professional help (reader, *please* learn from my mistake and seek help if you ever find yourself in a similar situation), and so never underwent any clinical assessment. What I do know is that combinations of acute stress and sleep deprivation (both of which I had a lot of at the time) are known to lead to hallucinations. As it turns out, loneliness is a highly prevalent experience in schizophrenia.[7] Maybe a combination of stress, loneliness, depression, sleeplessness and fatigue caused Jake and I to see things nobody else could. In other words, maybe they weren't real. I wonder how many people reading this book are saying "me too" right about now.

Another possible explanation is that people who experience chronic loneliness often scan for threats in their environment, even if subconsciously. Perhaps it is our brain's way of creating threats or stimuli because we are so deprived in our social isolation from actual threats, or making us see things that aren't there to encourage us to reconnect so we would feel safe again.

Interestingly, the hallucinations I experienced eventually ended once I reconnected and found meaningful friendships.

One of those new friends was a guy named Alan, who later stood beside me as a groomsman at my wedding. He said, "Joel, if you ever start seeing things again and it bothers you, call me. It doesn't matter if it's 3 o'clock in the morning, I will come over. You are not alone". The more friends like that I found in my life, the safer and happier I felt in this world. It felt *good* to know that someone out there cared for me.

Going back to my friend's story, I asked Jake if his psychiatrist had prescribed anything to help him manage his symptoms, and he shared that he was given Prozac, which he took for three years at the maximum dose he was legally allowed to take.

"What was that like, if you don't mind me asking? Did it help in any way?" I asked.

"Well, I didn't feel any better, nor did I feel worse, to be honest. It's like: say you're decelerating in a vehicle and you see the speed going down, slower and slower, to a point where it can stall and, just before it stalls, this medication comes in and throws you in neutral. You're not going any better, but you haven't stalled either."

"Oh really? That must have felt strange. I also heard that the medication can have side effects?"

"Yes, [it] did for me. I remember the first day of taking the medication very, very well. I felt like a zombie, fatigued as anything, barely walking, felt groggy. This was at school as well, so it didn't look too good in front of others. However, for the remainder of my time [taking] the medication, I've always described the feeling with one word: numb. Sure, you don't feel upset or sad, but you don't feel happy or energetic either. I was in this constant neutral, grey state of emotion for three years. It's as if the medication suppresses all emotion."

As someone who has never taken antidepressants, I found Jake's description intriguing. I would love to hear more stories from other people who are taking or have taken similar medication. As terribly numbing as it sounded, perhaps Prozac helped Jake from going downhill any further or saved him from hurting himself. I do acknowledge that antidepressants can be a greater help in some situations over others—that they may be effective in severe depression, but perhaps less so in mild depressive cases.

As our conversation drew to a close, I asked Jake if he had a close circle of friends now, living back in Australia. He said he had a few social circles, which was great, but none close enough for him to be able to open up to about his problems. I felt humbled that Jake felt safe enough to open up to me, but I am also hopeful that he continues to deepen his friendships with the right people and find other friends he can talk to in the near future. He is putting himself out there, getting exercise, helping others, and building his networks and connections. In even greater news, the relationship between Jake and his father is mending and they're growing closer than ever before. His dad used to frequently travel for work, but because of the pandemic, he's been working from home in Australia a lot more, enabling the two to eat and chat together more often at the family dinner table.

ADULTS

As we enter adulthood, many people experience new feelings of loneliness or social isolation to varying degrees, some of which are inevitable seasons in life's journey. In this section, I will share with you examples of situations that may affect our social connectedness and wellbeing as adults. My goal is to create awareness so not only can we, as individuals, take preventive measures, but also take part in reaching out to support others who might be feeling disconnected in their lives, at work, or in our community.

NEW MUMS

I was never deeply aware of post-natal depression until we had a glimpse of it when our first child was a few months old. Everything was going fine—at least I thought it was—until one day, Logan began to cry in his room. I was in our bedroom down the hall and called out to Belinda to see if she could check up on him, but she didn't respond. I called out a second time; perhaps she didn't hear me the first time. Again, she didn't respond. Meanwhile, Logan's cry grew louder and louder. I called out to Belinda for the third time and still heard no response, so I got up and searched for her, only to find her curled up, overwhelmed and in tears, on the living room couch. Seeing that she wasn't in a good place, I quickly ran to Logan's room to settle him in his cot. Once he was asleep, I went straight back to Belinda to check how she was going.

"Sorry ... I'm so so-rry," she said, stuttering through tears. I explained there was nothing to apologise for as I hugged and comforted her.

Later that night, I went online and started to read up on post-natal depression, trying to understand what my wife might be going through. What I learned, first of all, was that she was not alone in this. I discovered that all parents go through a period of adjustment as they try to manage the huge changes a baby brings into their lives. Belinda and I both experienced first-hand what it was like to wake up several times in the night to settle a crying baby back to sleep. You wake up the next day feeling so exhausted and sleep-deprived. Then, as I would head to work, Belinda would be left home alone with an infant, several days a week, who initially had trouble self-settling. While I got to interact with adults, Belinda often experienced the complete opposite as she didn't get to see or speak with other adults face-to-face—sometimes for the whole day—but was at least keeping in touch with friends by text or online. Her saving grace was when she could take Logan for a walk (for a while, a pram walk was the *only* way he would fall asleep) or catch up with the other mums in her weekly mother's group. She would sometimes get a visit from her parents or friends too, but there were many days she wouldn't see another adult until I came home from work.

I finally got a glimpse of what this feeling was like when I started parental leave. It can feel lonesome when you have no other adult to speak with for an entire day. I can't imagine how Belinda and so many other mums or dads do that full-time each and every day for an entire week, especially those who don't have family members or friends nearby to support them. Some days I wish it could be like life back home in the Philippines, where parents and grandparents live with you, while your neighbours come to say hi and check in with you from time to time. This means there's always someone there to keep you and the kids company. On top of that, live-in nannies are so affordable that most families have at least one, giving mums free time to do other things while the nannies take care of their children. It is undeniably true when they say it takes a village to raise a child but unfortunately, we just don't have this level of community in our Australian society. Sometimes we don't even know our own neighbours' names. We may say hi, but we don't make the effort to deepen our relationships unless they interest us. This culture of absolute privacy needs desperately to change, and it starts with you and me. *Of course* we need to be the change we want to see in the world.

NEW MIGRANTS

As part of a minority, first-generation migrants can face many challenges in the areas of language barriers, finances, jobs, community, networks and support, which combined can have a huge impact on mental health and social well-being. It's quite a significant topic when you consider that in 2020, nearly 30 percent of Australia's population were born overseas.[8]

It was 1991 and I was ten years old when my family of five arrived in Australia: my mum, Cora, my dad, Lito, and us three boys. Initially, we stayed with my mum's sister, 'Tita Mel', in Altona North, an industrial suburb 10 kilometres west of Melbourne, but she had a family of her own, plus her brother who lived with them. Add us into the mix and suddenly she had a full house of nine people with only three bedrooms and one bathroom to share. Space was cramped but we were thankful for the hospitality. A few months later, Dad met a man named David at a local church. He was a young Maltese guy in his twenties who had a kind face and happened to own a humble brick house just a few streets away from my aunt's place. He rented the house to us for only 100 dollars per week to help us out. It was old and cold but at least it was affordable and spacious, and it meant we could finally start out on our own as a family. Those early years were super tough on us, financially speaking, as my parents couldn't find any work. They weren't picky at all and would have gladly accepted any job offered to them but, unfortunately, the combination of us arriving on the back of a recession with little to no job coaching from anyone, language barriers, perhaps their age (being in their early forties) and no local experience or connections, all added up to making it very difficult for my parents to find employment.

Even though Dad was a barrister in the Philippines, it didn't help him here because he wasn't allowed to practice in the Australian legal system. He would have had to go back to university, but with no money in the bank and hungry mouths to feed, it wasn't really an option. Thankfully, being unemployed in Australia meant my parents got Social

Security payments from the government in the vicinity of around 600 dollars per fortnight, but that amount was barely enough to survive on. I don't know how families can live on 300 dollars a week. With rent, car and electricity bills to pay, groceries for five, medical, public school fees and other living expenses, there was never any savings left to spend on anything else. We had to be extremely frugal and only spend on necessities. It was a rude shock and a very difficult reality for us to adapt to.

I remember my eldest brother, Francis, saying to my dad, "Pa, why don't we just pack up and go home [to the Philippines]. We had everything we ever needed there, I had many friends and I was enjoying life. It hurts to see us suffer like this".

My dad replied, "Your mum and I never did this for us. We did it for you so you can have a better life. One day you will see. I promise". As noble as it sounded, it was fairly hard to comprehend or accept his foresight then, especially when we were living a hand-to-mouth existence.

Eventually, my dad found a volunteer job at a local migrant resource centre where he got to put his old accounting skills to good use (he was a certified practising accountant before becoming a lawyer) by helping out with their bookkeeping. The role not only kept him busy but also gave him purpose and a bit of local experience that he could put on his resume. Meanwhile, my mum continued to struggle to find a full-time job. Eventually, someone referred her to Adecco, a recruitment agency, which gave her casual work in factories from time to time. She would wait by the phone each morning hoping to receive a call from the agency to say she had a job that day, but more often than not she would not hear from them, which she found terribly depressing. I can imagine her being home alone, with no one to talk to, while dad went to work, and we kids went to school. That can be a pretty soul-destroying experience day after day for a migrant, especially when the call for work doesn't come. Years in this dead-end situation, with no money, and no close friends to talk with, mum felt detached and disconnected, which led to her loneliness, depression and mental health decline. Eventually, she displayed her frustrations by being aggressive toward us. Sometimes it was in the form of shouting or screaming. Other times she would resort to pinching or slapping me when she got mad about something—for example, if I didn't obey orders. One day, I came home from school and caught her in a really bad mood. I don't quite remember what I did that day that made her so mad, but she pulled me by the hair and slapped me hard across the face, causing my mouth to bleed. Her behaviour—verbal and physical abuse—continued for many years. She fell into a constant cycle of negative thinking. Not only was it damaging to her wellbeing, but it also impaired her relationships with her own family and friends, and perhaps even her ability to connect with society in general.

Fast forward to today and thankfully mum is a completely different person. If you met her now, you would say that she is a lovely woman and you wouldn't know any different. Upon reflection, I think it took 20 years for her to get to a happy place. Now, at retirement age, perhaps she has finally accepted her life in Australia. Maybe surviving breast cancer helped her get a new perspective of life, too. Or maybe it's the fact that all her children now have successful, stable careers and are married with beautiful children of their own, who she loves and adores. Whatever it is, I'm glad to see her in happier times and a better mental health state again. Despite the traumas I went through during her season of despair, I will always see mum as that beautiful, kind-hearted person who daily cooked us the most delicious foods, encouraged me in everything and supported me in taking risks in life. I will be forever grateful and never take for granted the sacrifices she and my dad made, just so we could live comfortably, safely, and happily as we do today.

This makes me think about all the other immigrants in Australia who are doing it tough at the moment, who are socially isolated, who are struggling to find employment, or who might be discriminated against. Many of them are silently suffering alone in their homes right now. I would know. Moving countries is like pulling a plant and its roots from its soil and replanting it somewhere else. An uprooted plant will benefit from as little trauma as possible when you water it, fertilise it and monitor its success. Similarly, if we set the example by welcoming migrants and helping them, showing them our tangible love and support, the sooner they can flourish, get on their own two feet and be productive and mentally healthier citizens. Not only would that be better for our economy, but we would enjoy a more connected and resilient society. I truly believe the answer to solving much of the loneliness and depression in our society is to help people to reconnect, and feel and know they belong.

ALONE IN A RELATIONSHIP

One thing many in our society sadly face is the prospect of feeling lonely in a relationship, particularly within a committed partner relationship, such as marriage. For one reason or another, couples who were once in love and deeply attentive to one another might begin to lose touch with one another's emotional needs, gradually growing apart, leaving one or both individuals feeling unhappy and alone in the relationship. In 2018, there were 119,188 new marriages in Australia, but also 49,404 divorces in the same year.[9] This is a staggering number, which is why I wanted to highlight this demographic here. Chances are you might know someone in your network going through this. Divorce—while sometimes the only feasible solution—not only impacts the couple but can have a ripple effect on their kids, their families and friends, their work and even the broader community at large. But, while staying unhappy isn't the only alternative in a relationship (yes, there *are* ways to re-establish your emotional connection)[10, 11], it's good to identify *why* we might find ourselves feeling alone to begin with—why we become emotionally distant.

According to the Australian Psychological Society, chronic relationship conflict and stress between partners is linked to poorer mental health and can negatively impact a person's other relationships with family, friends and colleagues.[12,13]

One of those impacts of an unhealthy marital or partner relationship is—you guessed it—loneliness, whether within the relationship itself or in one's broader network.

So, what are the major contributors when it comes to relationship problems? The Australian Psychological Society highlighted four factors:

PAST EXPERIENCES

Did you know your upbringing can heavily impact your future relationships? For example, people whose parents divorced or who witnessed high levels of conflict in the family home during their childhood are more likely to experience relationship problems later in life. Take a moment to consider your circumstances: has your relationship possibly been impacted by past experiences in your life or your partner's life? For one individual I interviewed, her upbringing had a particularly deep impact on her partner relationships. You will get to read Laura's story very soon.

LIFE TRANSITIONS AND STRESS

Imagine (or remember) getting married, moving in with somebody, having children and welcoming new in-laws into your life. Each of these life stages brings its own challenges, stresses and rewards. Moving to a new place or into a new job, experiencing work changes and setbacks, or coming into financial difficulties can all add to our life stresses and put a strain on our relationships.

I remember when Belinda and I faced our first serious financial stress after she had been on parental leave for

Logan. Month by month, our savings began to dwindle while Belinda looked for a new job. Small arguments would flare up as we began to feel the squeeze and found ourselves having to prioritise our spending more carefully (after years of living with a double income, no kids and very few financial worries). I'd heard many stories of couples arguing about money but, for the first time, we were experiencing it for ourselves. It was a deeply humbling experience, but one that fortified us in the end. The stresses of it would diminish every time I held my son or my wife (the power of a little oxytocin and perspective!). Belinda and I made a promise that as long as we were healthy and together as a family unit, we would never let money come between us. It wouldn't matter if we lost it all, we could rebuild as long as we were together. *That* is what's truly important.

HOW PEOPLE THINK

The 'lens' with which we view the world—ourselves, one another, our day-to-day lives—shapes the way we interpret words and situations, as well as our responses to them. This lens is influenced not only by culture (remember my chat with David from Hofstede Insights?) but also by our personalities and the broader collection of experiences we gather throughout life. When we come into a relationship with another human being, we often assume (consciously or subconsciously) that they're looking through the same lens as we are and often forget to explore and appreciate one another's unique perspectives. Sometimes it comes as a surprise then when our partner presents an entirely different view on a situation, and it can take time, openness and grace to choose to respond with humility instead of hurt.

For example, Belinda grew up in a white conservative Australian household. I was raised in a loud, expressive Filipino home. Belinda was trained in neuroscience and learned classical piano by graded syllabus. I'm more of a creative thinker and feeler and taught myself to play the guitar and write music. We met through our extended social networks and shared a common faith and love for the Philippines, but there was also a lot we didn't have in common. Some days it was like trying to connect a PC to a Mac. Our relationship got off to a rocky start when we first dated, but we soon realised the other person had very different ways of thinking about things. We learned to relax, and even compromise when we finally understood one another's perspectives.

Marriage certainly didn't make it any easier by itself or make our different ways of thinking go away, but it meant we invested more time in understanding and appreciating our differences. We read books like *His Needs, Her Needs* by Willard F. Harley, and *Love and Respect* by Emerson Eggerichs. We spent time seeing a professional who helped equip us with the right tools to build a solid marriage, and we joined our friends on a marriage retreat where we realised the things that tripped us up were the very same things that tripped up others.

Our marriage—far from perfect—has gotten better over time, but not by accident (no one ever drifted into a great marriage). It's a daily choice to love each other through our words and actions, remembering that we each think differently, choosing to invest in our personal growth, and continuing to fight for one another (all with a healthy dose of humour along the way), so neither of us feel alone.

BEHAVIOURAL FACTORS

Interactions that involve disrespect, criticism, defensiveness or stonewalling are behavioural signs that a relationship is at risk. Can you identify any of these signs that may have occurred regularly over the past four weeks in your own life? What happened and why? Are you able to come together with your partner to talk about the behaviours and explore the triggers or situations that lead to them, without leading to blame or shame of either person? Are there steps you can take to repair the relationship? Interestingly, it's been suggested that a ratio of five positive interactions to every one negative interaction with someone is a good indicator that your relationship is okay.

I hope these four factors have given you insight into some of the leading causes of relationship breakdown. In doing so, perhaps you can reflect and identify areas to work on to help restore your relationship(s) and avoid the sense of loneliness and disconnect that often accompanies chronic relationship stress. Don't hesitate to seek a professional counsellor or psychologist to help navigate conversations with your loved one and work through any of these areas. A great place to start could be to look up Australia Counselling or Relationships Australia to find a service near you.

❖ ❖ ❖

I will now introduce you to Laura, a divorcee who I recently interviewed for some insights into the causes of relationship breakdown. Laura's name has been changed to protect her identity.

To give you a little background, I first connected with Laura through church, but had not seen her in a long while before our chat, which I didn't think much of at the time—people often move away or find a new church to call home, which is a normal part of life. Then one day, I published a Facebook post looking to speak with people who were on antidepressant medication about their experiences and, to my surprise, Laura private-messaged me to say that she'd been taking antidepressants and would like to meet to share her story.

We met at a local café near her place. It was good to see Laura again—we hugged, sat down, and ordered pancakes and coffee (the ultimate rewards centre hit!). One thing I observed was how 'normal' Laura seemed, in that she appeared bubbly and energetic and was really happy to see me. To the outside world, you wouldn't have known she was struggling mentally. This goes to show how difficult it can be to determine how someone is feeling emotionally if we simply base it on their outward appearance—people can put on a brave face and smile even if they're feeling completely miserable.

"Joel, for you to understand the situation I am in, I would have to take you back to the very beginning," explained Laura.

"Sure," I replied.

"Okay, my father, who was the sole earner in the family, passed away when I was only nine years old. He drank a fair bit and eventually had a stroke and passed away. Mum didn't have a job so she had to pick herself up and take a full-time job in retail to feed four kids, of which I was the youngest.

"My journey with mental illness as a teenager came from not knowing how to ask for my needs to be met. I was lonely and attention-seeking but unfortunately Mum ignored my needs and simply told me to stop being silly. By age fifteen I was suicidal," Laura paused, perhaps to allow that bit of information to sink in.

"Oh," was the only thing I could think of saying in response.

I couldn't help but think of the impact her alcoholic father would have had on her as a child, and the impact his death had on the entire family; and, secondly, how her mother going to work would have meant spending less time at home with the kids, making it a real challenge for her to give them the appropriate share of her time, love and attention.

According to Collett Smart, psychologist and author of *They'll Be Okay* (a book for parents, which teaches them how to have conversations around uncomfortable but important topics with their children), parents' physical presence plays a very important role in their kids' development. Collett writes that "our children learn values from the adults they spend the most time with"[14] and that "one of the key factors that builds resilience in young people is a sense of being connected to adults".[15] She adds that "spending time with and meeting them where they are at is crucial to our children's healthy development".[16] According to Collett, there are positive associations for teens who spend an average of six hours a week engaged in family time with their parents ... if I may add—to feel loved, cared for, safe and supported. With Laura's father gone and a working mum, who she explains ignored her needs, no wonder she felt lonely and started seeking attention elsewhere.

I also want to highlight that there are always two sides to a story, and acknowledge that being a single parent is a tough job, let alone to four kids. I can only imagine what her mother's day-to-day would have been like: preparing the kids for the school day ahead, going to a job that perhaps she *needed* more than wanted, then coming home tired and still needing to prepare dinner for everyone, and once the kids are in bed, crashing on the couch, perhaps finding something to absorb her mind, to curb the loneliness of having no husband to talk to about her day. For those daily grinds that come with little to no help, I take my hat off to all single parents out there. Not only is it tough for the kids, but it is tough on you too.

By Year 12, Laura shared that her turning point was when two significant men made a positive impact in her life. The first was her English teacher, who she described as an encourager, and then a man named Mike, whom she met through a public speaking course she was doing. "He was a Christian (Protestant) and went to a local church. He knew I was raised Catholic but had been away from church, so he invited me along and I went. I was 17 at this point. I remember people asking me who I was and they remembered my name the next week when I came back. It was ground-breaking for me: they bothered to remember my name and what we talked about the previous week. This was a place where I could be part of a community," Laura's face was beaming as she spoke. I can just imagine how good it must have felt for her to be acknowledged, and how their conversations made her feel connected and listened to—something she had deeply longed for.

"That went well for a while, but I went back to my old habits as I still 'needed' a romantic relationship to feel valuable.

"Then I met someone who Mum liked, and we got married. I was 21 years old. He was not a Christian, so I gravitated away from the church to try to keep him happy. In a way, I made myself smaller for him to feel bigger but that meant I couldn't meet my needs. So, when after a few years I had to express myself again, he became aggressive. It came to a point where I had to leave to be safe, so I left him. I was 25 years old and I was divorced. I labelled myself 'unforgivable'. I then spent 18 months living alone going through panic attacks. I had this belief that I was not good enough and too sensitive, until one day I was sitting in my apartment, in the corner, having another panic attack because I couldn't remember which way to turn the door-knob to leave the house. I thought that the knob would fall off and I'd be stuck and no one would come to look for me, and I was going to starve to death. Thankfully, I had my phone and called my sister. She said, 'Stay where you are, I'll come and get you'.

"My sister finally came, and we went to a GP who prescribed Lexapro. I took it for years, although I didn't notice whether it helped or not. I trusted my GP, but I wasn't sure whether it was effective. That doctor then gave me a referral to see a psychologist who wasn't very helpful, so I went and saw two other psychologists who I didn't find useful either. Their approach was so clinical: I didn't understand why they were asking me to do certain things, for example, when I was having a panic attack," Laura said.

"What kind of things did they ask you to do?" I asked curiously.

"Well, they asked me to write down my thoughts and actions during my panic attack. They took the CBT [cognitive behavioural therapy] approach, which is an intervention strategy for unhelpful thinking. But I didn't have any distress tolerance skills, so the last thing I wanted to do was write down my thoughts, emotions and behaviours when I'm having a panic attack.

"So—I didn't find these guys particularly helpful, so I went into a mindset where nobody can help me. I tried therapy, which is quite expensive by the way, but nobody could help me, so I kept taking the medication until now. I've been taking them for close to 15 years. During that time, I've spent tens of thousands of dollars on doctors, psychiatrists, psychologists and antidepressants. Luckily, I have private [health] insurance. Without that, I would have paid hundreds of thousands and I'd be left penniless," Laura explained.

"That's a long time to be taking medications. How have they been for you?" I asked.

"Well, over the past 18 months, I've been getting lots of dry mouth, lockjaw, muscle tension, headaches, nose bleeds, nausea and weight gain," she answered. "Some products give me a feeling of unreality, where [I'd] sit there and sense the distance of the stars and planets, or I'd be walking in the street and everything feels so close to me, while other brands keep me alert, so I can't take them after lunchtime otherwise I can't go to sleep."

I just sat there and listened. It was a lot to take in and process.

Laura said taking antidepressants wasn't the final answer for her but, for now, it's part of the solution. My time with her was coming to a close and I used those last few minutes to encourage her to seek community again and to find ways to reconnect for her own mental and social wellbeing. Laura married a second time but, unfortunately, was in the process of going through her second divorce when we caught up. She told me that she was only discharged from the hospital a week earlier as she'd felt like taking her own life.

I felt helpless for Laura and guilty for going our separate ways knowing full well that she wasn't in a good place. It made me wonder how things may have played out if her father had not been an alcoholic and was still alive today. Collett explains in her book that "when a daughter has a secure, supportive and communicative relationship with her dad, she is more likely to create and maintain emotionally intimate, fulfilling relationships with men" and that "a close relationship with Dad can lead to daughters being more assertive and self-confident in refusing to have sex when they do not wish to, as well as refusing to be emotionally dominated by their partners".[17] Lastly, Collett writes that absent fathers create a gaping emotional need for belonging and acceptance in children that the children try to fill in other ways, such as sex, drugs and alcohol. Laura's story is a complicated one. I hope it gives you an awareness of how someone might feel alone in a relationship, the contributing factors and the mental health challenges that come with it. If you know anyone on the verge of a relationship breakdown or divorce or know a single parent, please do reach out, ask how they are and be prepared to listen to their answer. Your call could be the best thing that happened to them today.

LONELINESS IN THE WORKPLACE

Local research has shown that a large number of Aussie workers across the country feel lonely in the workplace, which has an alarming impact on their productivity and general wellbeing. If you've ever felt lonely at work, then you know that sense of being surrounded by people, yet feeling completely alone.

According to the 2019 Workplace Loneliness report by Reventure, 40 percent of Australian workers have felt lonely or somewhat lonely at work in the past 12 months.[18] Headed by Melbourne-based Dr Lindsay McMillan, the survey was completed by a nationally representative sample of 1,010 employed Australians between 18 to 65 years, of which 62 percent of respondents were workers, and 38 percent employers, which included owners and managers.

The report also showed that feelings of loneliness in the workplace cause a number of damaging flow-on effects: workers experiencing loneliness are twice as likely to look for a new job; 49 percent of Australian workers who have experienced workplace loneliness say they are more likely to withdraw from their colleagues; 47 percent report their overall wellbeing suffers; and 46 percent became less engaged with the workplace vision and values. In terms of work performance, 40 percent of lonely workers said they felt less productive, while 38 percent reported they were more likely to make mistakes at work or get sick (36 percent).

We spend most of our daily lives working—whether on-site or from home—and I believe if we don't start intentionally creating deeper, genuine connections with the people around us, then we risk having only transactional relationships with our staff and colleagues, which will almost certainly lead to feelings of loneliness, isolation and unhappiness in the workplace.

According to a survey of 200,000 people around the world by Boston Consulting Group, two of the top four factors for employee happiness are not related to a bigger salary, but rather—drum roll please—good relationships with colleagues and superiors, and being appreciated for one's work.[19] Let's reflect on that for a second. I think this speaks volumes about what people really crave: healthy connections. It makes total sense. Underneath all the clothes, titles or how much we earn, we all share that primitive, basic human need as social beings. Together, this survey and the Workplace Loneliness report highlight just how critical it is for organisational leaders to listen and act to create environments and cultures that emphasise meaningful connections, otherwise expect to face the dire effects that loneliness has on both the employee and the company itself.

So, what's causing loneliness in the workplace? I'll try to highlight some real-life examples here that I've come across in my network and my own lived experiences.

One contributing factor is technology itself—online communication tools, in particular, which include voice, video or messaging capabilities. While such technologies have drastically improved real-time interactions, they can also inhibit us from fostering meaningful face-to-face human connections with one another. I remember the good old days when we used to walk up to each other to talk. Nowadays, we email or instant message our colleagues to strike up a conversation or ask a question. As I touched on in Chapter 6, I'm guilty of this practice myself. Only the other day, I found myself instant-messaging two of my colleagues using Microsoft Teams who were both sitting right next to me. One of them, Steve, quickly laughed when he saw it and said, "I'm right next to you". I was embarrassed, of course, and sheepishly laughed it off. Still, many people prefer to use digital communication tools believing they are more efficient than speaking in person. However, much of our communication is non-verbal, such as our facial expression, tone of voice and body language. We lose all of this on emails and text, which can sometimes lead to misunderstandings. More importantly, it fails to provide the social interactions we need as human beings.

Recently, I surveyed my network to share their thoughts and experiences on factors that can lead to feelings of loneliness and social isolation in the workplace. I've changed their names for anonymity.

Chris, who once worked at a growing tech start-up said, "The amount of travel I had with my previous company left me quite isolated. It made me feel like I was a contractor, not like I was part of the team. Home life was massively impacted too. Not only was I present just three days a week, but a by-product of high travel was it made me very comfortable with my own company. I don't think it's generally a bad thing but not good when I get back home and try to be involved with my wife and kids". Despite his good salary, Chris resigned from that company as a result.

Paul, who works as an international flight attendant said, "The topic of loneliness affects those in my industry in a huge manner that is unseen and undetected by the general public. The usual flight attendant is seen as well-presented and charming because of that plastered-on smile, and happy because of the work they are doing and the chance of a great time at their destination. However, the opposite rings true to quite a lot of us. The walls of the hotel rooms we've stayed in have heard our cries and felt our disconnections".

Deb, who works in a publishing company said, "I get stressed and lonely at work because they put us together with tech people who only chat to each other by computer. We are not allowed to even giggle or have a verbal conversation. I don't think you can really combine artists and tech people in one room. Technology really makes us like robots".

Then, Tom, who works for a big-four accounting firm said, "I have 100 percent felt lonely over the last year working on client sites for long periods of time either by myself or with colleagues who tend not to engage in 'out-of-work chat'. [It] can be pretty tough when the client hides you in a meeting room and you feel you have no one to talk to. Then walking into a full bustling client kitchen and being the odd one out sucks".

Who you are outside of work matters too. The higher the quality of the relationships you have in your private life, the better you become at keeping loneliness at bay.

Melanie, who works in telco said, "I almost never socialise at work and I choose to work from home rather than go in when I can (I'm just more productive at home) but I think it's because I have other communities, such as church. Although, I don't know how I'd be if I did not have those other networks. This just makes me value my community even more".

Another friend, Jim, who is a director for a bank said, "I don't socialise much with co-workers but only because I have other communities. I do find that when I was working overseas and had no usual network, the workplace was the only way I could make friends".

It appears that loneliness can affect anyone from any sector, but according to Betterup, which conducted a survey with American workers to identify those employees most at risk for feeling lonely at work, some workplaces are lonelier than others. In a breakdown of loneliness and social support rates by profession, they found lawyers to be the loneliest, followed by engineers, then those who work in the field of science.[20]

Meanwhile, in Australia, medicine appears to be one of the loneliest and most stressful fields, at least according to Australia's first Chief Medical Wellness Officer, Dr Bethan Richards, who is based at Sydney Local Health District. With suicide rates 120 percent higher for female doctors than the general public and 40 percent higher for males, people outside the field still don't truly understand what the problem is, and that it's an epidemic happening in the medical field globally, not just here.

Introduced through a mutual friend, I caught up with Dr Richards at a café near the Royal Prince Alfred Hospital to hear her story.

"Call me Bethan," she said.

Bethan looked to be in her late thirties and reminded me of the actress, Jodie Foster, with her mid-length light brown hair and the way she talked a little husky.

"Could you tell me a bit about how you came into the role?" I asked.

"Sure. When I became a director of medical training for medical registrars [junior doctors], I began to see the struggles these trainees go through, which become more intense and stressful as their years of study progress. They were suffering and I wanted to understand why. During that time three suicides happened. This gave me the motivation I needed to do something about it. I went back to the evidence and looked at wellbeing programs and saw one, which was based on a Stanford Medicine model, which focuses on principles and applications that contribute to physician wellbeing. I then completed a course studying this model in the US. This eventually led to the creation of my (additional) role as chief medical wellness officer for SLHD."

"So, it's been six months into your role. What kind of activities have you put in place?" I asked.

"Well, some of the base stuff in the program include exercise and yoga, but the social part is what we added this year. It's the thing that everyone is yearning for as these specialists are siloed. So, part of what I'm proposing is to put a staff lounge for everyone, so that doctors and nurses alike can socially interact and get to know one another," she explained.

Bethan also observed that more senior doctors were also distressed, burned out, anxious and depressed. "About 30 percent of my colleagues are going through burnout, so one of the things we are introducing is uninterrupted lunch breaks between 12 to 1 pm so they can have lunch. These are protected lunch breaks where no one can send a call-out to the doctor." Bethan went on to share that many of her peers would skip their meal breaks because they felt obliged to put their patients' needs first.

It is early days, but I am glad to see people like Bethan, who are making a difference in their workplace, especially one as challenging as the frontline of healthcare. Her ultimate goal is to be able to go back to Canberra to talk with our government and say, "Hey, the program is working. If we can do it to a place like this (Sydney Local Health District has 14,000 employees), we can do it somewhere else". I can't wait to speak with her again over the next two to three years to hear the outcome of her wellness program and how it's impacting both physicians' lives and their patients in a positive way.

FREELANCE WORK

Another workplace trend that may be a contributing factor to loneliness now and into the future is freelance work. Some call it the 'gig economy' or perhaps more appropriately the 'on-demand economy'. These are individuals who engage in temporary, supplemental, project or contract-based work. Think of work-from-home jobs such as digital marketing, web development, graphic design, mobile app development or photography. Some freelance work involves working on-demand in different places or on-the-go. You may have even dabbled in this space as an Uber or Deliveroo driver, or perhaps as an Airtasker, where you bid to complete tasks outsourced by people in your community.

According to the 2017 Freelancing in America survey conducted by Edelman Intelligence, if freelancing continues to grow at its current rate, 50 percent of the US workforce will be freelancing by 2027.[21] Digital platforms such as Airtasker, Uber or Freelancer.com are making it easier for people to find on-demand work these days, with Australians also joining the freelance revolution in rising numbers. An Australian survey of more than 14,000 people commissioned by the Victorian Government in 2019 found that 7.1 percent of those surveyed were working through a digital platform or had done so in the past 12 months.[22] While that number may sound like a small proportion of our entire workforce, the probability of that number growing is high, if the US sector is anything to go by. Though I'm sure the gig economy can bring about benefits and rewards for the individual and our broader economy, I can't help but think about the potential mental health implications it poses for freelancers.

For example, according to the Victorian Government survey, the majority of Aussie freelancers are working from home (55.3 percent). Considering many of us are already feeling lonely in the workplace, even when we are surrounded by people, I wonder how much more isolated we might feel when we are working remotely with no face-to-face contact throughout the day? While the idea of sending emails in your pyjamas may sound appealing, working as a freelancer may come at a cost. For some of us, it can even put our mental health at risk. Social isolation can make us vulnerable in the gig economy where there is a lack of social integration. In comparison to a more stable permanent job, those in precarious employment (such as temporary, seasonal or casual employment) may show lower levels of connectedness or belonging.

Knowing that this work trend will continue to grow into the future, I would predict that reports of loneliness over time will begin to surface and likely increase in proportion to the number of people joining the gig economy. If so, we need to start preparing now and think about social isolation preventative measures in this line of industry, as well as educating and instilling lifestyle practices that help freelancers to stay connected with their family, friends and the general community, to help build their resilience against the risks of chronic loneliness and/or depression.

WORKING FROM HOME DUE TO COVID-19

Interestingly, as I write this book, much of the entire world is practising physical distancing by working from home due to COVID-19. Companies like Twitter, Facebook, Atlassian, even Google and Microsoft are inviting their employees to do this indefinitely or permanently. But the question is, are we emotionally ready? In a way, we are all taking part in the biggest social experiment in history and are experiencing first-hand what it might be like to work remotely, along with the associated impacts on our mental health. Calls to Lifeline Australia have already jumped by 20 percent in 2020, which doesn't come as a surprise. I predict that mental health service providers worldwide will also report overwhelming increases in demand as people seek mental help to overcome the stresses that have surfaced during their lockdowns and periods of isolation. I find it ironic that I'm writing a book on social wellbeing at a time when we are being asked to physically distance ourselves from others. As our governments tell us to stay in our homes to help control the spread of COVID-19, socially connecting ourselves has become a very important topic now more than ever.

We all know by now the benefits of working from home—you know, saving two hours of public transport each day and the ability to create more memories with the family—but, sadly, there are also hidden costs that we need to be aware of, especially for those of us who live alone. When we're inside the house in lockdown for prolonged periods, away from nature, away from friends, we start to become disconnected—some of us more than others. And, when we don't have other people to bounce our ideas off or spend meaningful time with, we can start to lose our ability to self-regulate, which is a critical building block of resilience that involves controlling one's behaviour, emotions and thoughts.

One of my biggest concerns at the moment is that too many organisations have not yet designed any thorough framework, guidelines or checklists on how their staff can look after their wellbeing as they work from home. COVID-19 is such a new situation that many employers have not fully considered or understood the potential ramifications of this move.

I shared earlier that even before COVID-19, 40 percent of Australian workers already felt lonely at work, with 38 percent of lonely workers making more mistakes, and 40 percent of lonely workers feeling less productive. Can you imagine what loneliness and staff productivity statistics will look like in 12 months' time, now that we are working remotely and have less social contact than ever before? We used to see people on the bus, socialise with colleagues in the office, catch up with friends during lunch breaks or meet clients during the week. But COVID-19 took away most of that. Surely this can only increase feelings of loneliness in employees, along with anxiety and depression.

When we're lonely, our wellbeing suffers. When our wellbeing suffers, our whole being suffers: our productivity and creativity suffer, we become more prone to mistakes and illness, and we become unhappy. But these things don't only affect the individual, they affect their business, their families and those around them too, including peers and colleagues. We spend the majority of our waking hours each week at work. Ultimately, employers have a duty of care to look after the wellbeing of employees, and I would urge them that *now* is the time to implement a holistic program that fosters not just their mental, physical or financial health, but their social connections too, and integrate it into the overall strategy of their organisation, regardless of whether employees work in the office, remotely or a combination of both.

❖ ❖ ❖

In this chapter, I have shared some examples of groups of people who are particularly vulnerable to loneliness and the subsequent mental health problems that can follow when their needs—particularly social wellbeing needs—are not met. In the next chapter, we will focus on the practical ways we can keep loneliness at bay, manage social isolation, and I include tips for how to reconnect to stay physically, mentally and socially healthier. ❖

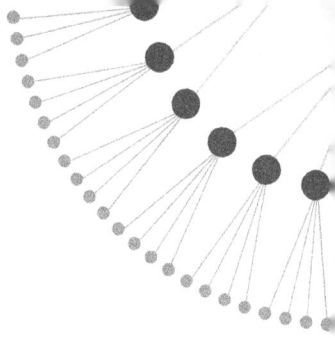

CHAPTER 7

How Can I Build New Connections?

Remember, in the words of Dr Michelle Lim, "Acute loneliness is okay, but we must absolutely treat chronic loneliness" because it leads to a wide range of negative and crippling effects on our mental health. Compounding this, COVID-19 has caused even greater concern for those of us who have become more susceptible to prolonged feelings of loneliness and isolation due to snap lockdowns, physical distancing measures and border restrictions. As COVID-19 spreads throughout the modern world, killing millions of people and infecting hundreds of millions more, governments everywhere are introducing laws preventing people from leaving their homes unless absolutely necessary, with the objective of controlling the spread.

One of the downsides of these measures is that they've caused many of us to feel more disconnected than ever before. This may not affect everyone in the same way, or even to the same extent but I desperately need to get out of the house every now and then to stay sane—whether it be to exercise, see nature or catch up with friends. During the early months of the pandemic, I had to work from home for a few weeks straight and, I must say, it was a strange feeling to have suddenly stayed indoors for this prolonged period of time. Luckily for me, my wife Belinda was also working from home, so I at least had someone to talk with. I can't help but wonder how this current state of play could be impacting the wellbeing of those who live alone. While phone and video calls help us stay connected, nothing beats that all-important face-to-face contact. In her TEDx talk 'The secret to living longer may be your social life'[1], Susan Pinker explains how digital interaction is not the same as interacting in person: "Face-to-face contact releases a whole cascade of neurotransmitters … simply making eye contact with somebody, shaking hands, giving somebody a high-five, is enough to release oxytocin, which increases your level of trust, and it lowers your cortisol levels, so it lowers your stress. And dopamine is generated, which gives us a little high and it kills pain. It's like a naturally-produced morphine".

So, if you've ever wondered why it generally feels better seeing a friend or close colleague in person, you now have the scientific evidence to explain the physiology behind it. In a world where technology has allowed us to connect faster and more efficiently with others across vast distances, it turns out the secret to building better relationships and possibly living longer and healthier lives could be as simple as seeing people the old-fashioned way: *in person.*

Now that we've all experienced a degree of social isolation and physical distancing as a result of COVID-19 and felt first-hand what that does to our wellbeing, would you agree that we should make a conscious effort to reconnect and *stay intentionally connected* with friends, family and our community? If so, let's have a closer look at our social layers.

YOUR CIRCLES OF FRIENDS

As much as we need social contact, we can't be best friends with everybody. It's simply not possible to invest your time equally with everyone in your circles: you end up spreading yourself too thin and burning out in the process. You may have 700 Facebook friends but your closest friends—the ones you enjoy investing time in—may just be a handful. Your circles of friends can be best described in the diagram below. The smallest circle is your 'inner circle' of trust. The middle circle encompasses your 'social friends'.

And the outermost circle is defined by your 'broader community'. The closer you get to the inner circle, the deeper and more meaningful your connections will be with those people.

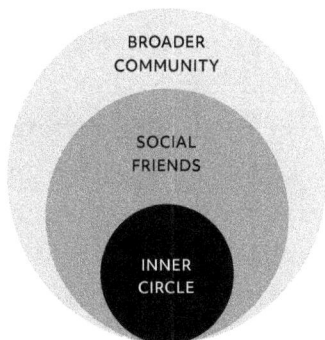

YOUR BROADER COMMUNITY

This group of acquaintances you've built over time may number in the hundreds (maybe more, maybe less), depending on your age, what you do, where you live and your personality. This circle is characterised by the lowest degree of trust. For example, they could be the librarian you borrow books from, a business channel partner or the personal trainer at the gym you go to. It could also be your doctor, your mechanic or maybe your kid's piano teacher. You've met them a few times, so you would know their names.

YOUR SOCIAL FRIENDS

This group contains a level of trust in the relationship but not as much as your inner circle. This group may contain 20 to 40 people and you see these people often throughout the year. You know them enough that they become people you end up going to parties, the beach or a concert with or have lunches or dinners with. You're comfortable in their company. They might include your classmates, your friends from team sports, your work colleagues, friends from shared religious or spiritual communities, people from your parenting group or even your close neighbours. Your social friends will introduce you to business connections. They'll even help you move house or give you a place to stay for the night. Some may even make you meals if you've just had a baby, as was the case for us after Logan was born. It's humbling to have friends like these who can be so generous with their time, money and service when the need arises.

YOUR INNER CIRCLE

These are your closest connections. They're generally around three to five people who you can share anything with and trust with your deepest secrets. They are the people you share the most meaningful connections with. They could be your spouse, family and best friends. These are people you can call at any time of day and will be there for you and have your back but are also there to hold you accountable and tell you the truth. As the saying goes: "True friends say good things behind your back and bad things to your face". They want to see you grow and succeed in life. Your closest friends want the best for you, even if it means having the tough conversations.

These three groups are important to your social and mental health to varying degrees and for various reasons. People can also track across, or in and out of these circles in different seasons—your 'lines' between circles may appear more like dynamic gradients, especially between the two outer circles. Even so, we all need a solid social network. Our circles of friends are there to support us and reciprocally, we are there to support them. Not only do we need these relationships in the good times, but we especially need them in times of loneliness, depression or crisis, as we are all undoubtedly experiencing while being asked to stay home and physically distance ourselves from others during the pandemic.

BUILDING MY PERSONAL COMMUNITY

I'm going to share a few suggestions about how you can build your own circles of friends. But before I do, let me tell you the story of how I came to build mine by coming to church. This isn't to say that religious or spiritual communities are the only option for people to build their circles up, but I am sharing that it was the foundation that worked for me.

If you remember from earlier chapters, I shared how my personal struggle with chronic loneliness and depression led me to move from Melbourne to Sydney. The hard thing about moving to a new place is that you often have zero friends to begin with. Despite or perhaps because of this, my move to Sydney became a blessing in disguise, as it gave me the opportunity to start with a clean slate and the freedom to choose the friends I wanted to bring into my world.

I'm sure you would appreciate this is easier said than done. For starters, it can sometimes feel uncomfortable to meet new people (that's still often the case for me) and it also takes a lot of effort. To meet people, you have to be intentional. New friends don't just appear on your front door and say, "Hey, I want to be your friend, may I come in?" You *must* put yourself out there to meet them—and more than once, twice or three times!

Of all places, the opportunity to find and build my new community started one fine summer morning when my radio alarm went off, playing 2GB with Alan Jones. Yes, I was that 25-year-old who listened to Alan Jones every day. I woke up listening to him this particular morning as he interviewed a young woman in a conversation that led me to a community that would change my life forever. No matter what people think of Alan Jones, you could say his interview that day became the catalyst that helped me to meet the circle of friends I have today.

"So, tell me about yourself. Your music reached the number one spot in the ARIA music charts, yet most Australians probably wouldn't know who you guys are. Please tell our viewers your name and tell us a bit about your group," Alan asked the young woman.

"Thanks for having me, Alan. Hi, everyone. My name is Brooke Fraser and I'm part of the worship team at Hillsong. We're a group of people who catch up, write songs and sing Christian-based music. Everyone is welcome to come along and check it out," she said.

There was something about her that seemed warm, friendly and inviting. I thought to myself, "Hey, I'm a musician, a singer and a guitar player, too. We have something in common. Maybe I should check it out and watch them in one of their jam sessions. They seem like the type of people I'd like to get to know. After all, she said I'd be welcome". Plus, it was a brand-new year. I thought it would be great to kick it off meeting new people: a brand-new start.

As a quick fact, Brooke Fraser is an accomplished and talented New Zealand-based singer-songwriter who, by the age of 18, was snapped up by Sony Music. Her music has topped the charts several times both in her native country of New Zealand and here in Australia.

As silly as it may sound, I initially took the syllables 'hill' and 'song' quite literally and presumed that Brooke and her friends played music up on a hill somewhere! I looked up where to go and off I went one Saturday afternoon in January 2007 to find these musicians on a hill.

"You must be Joel. Welcome to Hillsong," said Andi Andrew, a woman in her late twenties with long, brown wavy hair and a disarming smile. I had emailed them a week earlier and said I would be visiting but that I didn't know anyone there, which made me a little apprehensive. Andi, who was part of the Hillsong team, had emailed me back to say there was nothing to worry about and that she'd be more than happy to welcome me herself when I arrived at their Waterloo location. After our brief introduction, Andi ushered me in to take a seat. I looked around and it wasn't anything like what I expected. I thought I'd be watching some musicians in a room. But this was bigger—it was an auditorium filled with seats, with maybe 300 people in the crowd. In front of us was a stage, like what you'd see in a high school hall. While background music played, I could see people chattering away with friends, saying hello to strangers or giving hugs to people they knew. I sat there, observing, patiently waiting for something to begin, though I didn't know what exactly or when.

Then suddenly, the stage lights turned on and a guy holding a guitar welcomed the crowd, a band now playing behind him as he began to sing, and the audience started to sing along with him. Some were reading lyrics from a big screen right in front of us, while others, eyes closed, sang the lyrics off by heart. The band was playing so well—too well, I thought. Am I at a concert? No. This was a free event. It was a full band—there were people playing the drums, keys, bass and an acoustic guitar and the singer was vocally excellent. It was impressive. The best way I could describe it was they sounded more like a group you'd hear on Australia's Top 40. No wonder they had topped the charts as Alan had described. Their music was upbeat, uplifting and catchy. It certainly wasn't something I expected to hear. I could see how this contemporary Christian music would connect and appeal to a younger audience. As I looked around, I could see the place was filled mostly—but not entirely—with young adults, from late teens to those in their thirties. They were in my age group, which I found fascinating.

Growing up in a Catholic family, I was always forced to go to Mass with my parents, with very little choice in the matter. It was *not* cool and I was *never* willing. My father used to get upset when I'd tell him I couldn't go. There was never a good enough excuse to not come to church with him.

Me: Dad, I'm sick.

Dad: Joel, get in the car.

Me: Dad, I didn't sleep well last night.

Dad: That's your problem. Get in the car.

Me: Dad, I need to study for my exams.

Dad: So? It's only an hour of your time each week. Get in the car.

The truth was, I found going to Mass every Sunday morning as a kid and teenager mind-numbingly boring. It was the same ritual every week and I didn't feel like I was learning anything—it didn't connect with my heart or my mind, let alone my soul. I only ever went to make my dad happy, and that was that. But here, in this other church I found myself in, the young adults were here out of their own free will. They seemed to be really enjoying themselves, even loving it.

I looked back to the stage. I couldn't sing along because I'd never heard these songs before but I found myself tapping my foot to the rhythm. Some people even had their hands up in the air, singing so passionately. I couldn't process what was happening around me because it was so foreign and strange and it all happened so fast. I was overwhelmed but by now I was beginning to understand how music like this could both top the charts and win the soul. It sounded great and it felt different.

After a set of songs, a guy walked on stage and welcomed the crowd, "Hello church. Happy New Year. My name is Nick Khiroya, I'm one of the pastors here at church". He looked quite young to be a pastor, I thought. Based on my Catholic experiences, priests were generally much older and wore long white garments from the neck down with a long red scarf. But Nick must have been in his mid-twenties and wore sneakers, a t-shirt and jeans. He had freshly cut short black hair. He appeared easy-going, confident and well-spoken.

Nick then proceeded to preach for the next half an hour, and the service ended with a final song. By that time, I knew I had found myself a place to call home—spiritually and socially. Something shifted inside of me that night, and I could tell my life was finally heading on a new trajectory.

At the end of the service, some people went home; some went to dinner together; others stayed back to hang out with friends or connect with new ones. Apart from Andi, I met three more people that evening who each approached me separately after the service and introduced themselves. Simon, Rebecca and Michael were their names and I'm proud to say I'm still connected with them today after all these years. Simon has even become a good friend of mine, and I was the photographer at Michael's wedding.

These three people said things like: "Welcome to church, Joel"; "Great to meet you. Is this your first time visiting us?"; "Which part of Sydney are you from?"; and "I look forward to seeing you again, maybe?"

Everyone was so kind and non-confronting in their approach, which made me feel relaxed and comfortable. After spending one and a half years alone in Sydney, it was great to finally engage in a social conversation with people other than my work colleagues. I felt genuinely welcomed, which made me want to come back, partly because I wanted to learn more about Christianity, but also because I hadn't felt so accepted in such a long time. I didn't feel lonely for once. I remember heading home feeling happy and invigorated. I knew at that point that it would be a year of new beginnings.

I went back the following week. As I entered the foyer, I suddenly felt the urge to pick up one of the welcome card baskets and start handing cards out to people coming inside the church.

"Hi, I don't think I've seen you around here before. Are you part of our welcome team?" asked one of the church staff.

"No," I answered, "I'm fairly new here. I came last week for the first time. People were so welcoming to me that I now want to do the same and welcome others too".

"Wow, you're awesome! Don't let me stop you. Welcome away." She went back to the front desk, looked over at her colleague and pointed at me, both of them smiling from ear to ear.

From then on, I met even more people by joining a 'connect group'—a gathering of about six to twelve people within the church who meet regularly to establish a sense of community, catch up and do life together. With so many people coming to church, someone like me could easily get lost in the crowd and not establish a relationship with anyone at a deeper level. This, I learned, is where connect groups play a vital role.

Let me explain how. I remember being introduced to my first connect group in Manly, in the Northern Beaches of Sydney where I was residing at the time. A beautiful young couple named Sara and Ramon ran the group. Ramon worked in IT security and Sara was a midwife. Everyone in our group was in their late twenties or early thirties, and since we all worked in professional full-time jobs, we met up at the Buckland's place every second Tuesday night after work, where we each got to share how life was going. It was like coming home from school or work, where your family asks how your day went. It was a safe place where you could be vulnerable and share your highs and lows; where you could encourage, support and challenge one another, and keep each other accountable. Surrounding myself with these people of good character not only helped me to see things from different perspectives, but it helped me to grow and develop my character as well.

In addition to our fortnightly meet-ups, some of us would get together casually over coffee, lunch or dinner during the week. On weekends, we would sometimes meet by the beach and hang out. The more contact we had, the closer and more comfortable we got with one another. The group became my instant family away from home. I never felt judged but instead accepted for who I was and nurtured to grow. It didn't matter what nationality I was, where I came from, what I did or whether I was well-off or penniless. Reflecting on it now, I consider myself very fortunate to have been part of this group of people at that point in my young adult life. I *needed* it for building my mental health and resilience against the day-to-day stressors and challenges in life.

By embedding myself into this micro-community, I began to experience first-hand and learn how to treat people better, and how to go above and beyond for others through the little things my connect group did that made me feel like I belonged and was cared for and listened to.

Let me share an example. One morning, I was on my way to work on the ferry from Manly to Circular Quay, when Ramon called unexpectedly. "Hey Joel, it's Ramon. How are you going?"

"I'm doing good, man. Is everything alright?" I asked.

"Yeah, everything's well," Ramon replied, "I was just thinking of you, so I thought to give you a call and say hi".

"Oh, okay," I said, feeling unsure of what to say next.

Luckily, Ramon easily filled in the gaps and started talking, so we continued with the chat for another five to ten minutes. I hung up and thought to myself that I don't remember *anyone* ever doing that for me before. The call made me feel valued. Because of Ramon leading by example, I've been checking up on others ever since.

Challenge time: Why don't you surprise-call someone this week? Why not right now? Unless you haven't called your parents in a long time, the challenge is to call someone other than an immediate family member. Maybe it's an old friend or an acquaintance—or maybe a new friend! Say you've been thinking about them and go from there. It's okay to check in on people without an agenda. That call will have a lasting impact on them, I promise.

Back to my story: I continued going to church every weekend (which, it turns out, *wasn't* located on a hill, despite its name!) and making the constant decision to meet more people. Hillsong felt a bit like the United Nations because it was a melting pot of people from all parts of the world—such as Brazil, Africa, America, Canada, Asia and Europe—and it gave me the privilege to learn and appreciate all of my new-found friends' cultures. Everyone from doctors, lawyers, carpenters, accountants, scientists, psychologists—people in all sorts of careers—were there. Broadly speaking, I don't think you could find any other place where you get this kind of exposure to people from all walks of life other than in church. I've heard it said that we fear what we don't understand; and yet here I was immersing myself, appreciating people not only for who they were, but where they came from—fear had no place in this community.

Something I soon realised I had in common with many of these people was that we all came from interstate or overseas and, in a way, we were all searching for some kind of community outside our workplace. The more I turned up, the more people I got to meet, and the more friends and connections I was able to make. It had felt like only yesterday that I didn't have anyone to talk to and was all alone in the world. And now I was meeting lots of people in this community, like a fountain of new and meaningful relationships had erupted and overflown, washing over my memories of loneliness.

Now, I completely understand if church isn't your thing. There are other ways of making friends that you may be more comfortable with. Let's have a look at some of them now.

MY TOP THREE WAYS TO BUILD YOUR OWN COMMUNITY

I've been waiting eagerly to share this with you. *This* is where the fun begins—the world is your oyster when it comes to meeting people. The key is, you *must* give it a go—and *keep* giving it a go. People won't know you exist unless you put yourself out there. You need to be completely invested and intentional in meeting others for this to work, and it doesn't matter whether you're an introvert, extrovert or somewhere in the middle (ambivert).

Interestingly, many of my friends would tell you I'm an extrovert but I'm actually more leaning towards being introverted. They'd say I'm like a ball of energy when I'm around people but the truth is I choose to put the extra effort into socialising. As a result of this extra effort, I generally feel drained from it and need alone time afterwards to recharge my batteries, which is unlike my extroverted wife who confounds me with the way she is so utterly energised from being around people.

If you build the foundation now, where you create a community around you and find people who will be there to support you during times of crisis—to lend you a shoulder to cry on—you *will* have better mental health. If you can find friends to play, laugh or cry with; friends who will want the best for you and not to harm you; friends who will lift you up and speak life into you, you will find a new source of strength, a new source of confidence, and a new source of happiness that you've never experienced before.

Many years ago, an acquaintance asked me, "Joel, where do you get your confidence from? Your joy is infectious". It was the first time anybody had said that about me.

I remember pointing behind me when I replied, "There are hundreds of people watching out for me. They aren't here right now but I have these friends who want the best for me, friends who help me be a better version of myself today, friends who wish me all the success and happiness in life. In times of need or crisis, I can make a call and they will come to my aid. If I need a place to stay anywhere in the world, chances are I will know someone who lives there and they'll be more than happy to open their homes up to me. So, you see, even though they aren't physically here with me, I know I've got people in my life who have my back and that brings me great joy".

As you know, going to church was the building block for me in establishing this great network. "But Joel, I'm not the churchy kind. It's really not for me," you might say. Thankfully, there are *so* many other ways to build your community, your tribe. If that's what you're after, let's have a look at a few ideas now to get you started. You might want to grab some tea or coffee because this section is for you to work through slowly, not simply breeze through. Let's begin.

1. ATTEND AN INTEREST GROUP

Is there something you're passionate about or that piques your interest but you have never tried? This could be a great place to start. Maybe you're into sports, music, arts, reading, dancing, cycling, walking, cars, politics, photography … or anything else. It doesn't have to cost you anything to be in a group or social club with people who have similar interests.

For example, Meetup.com is a service used to organise in-person events for people with similar interests. This is how it works:

Step 1: Find a group on the website
Step 2: Check out their event dates

Step 3: Confirm your attendance and go

It's that simple. Don't worry if you don't know anyone there at first. Chances are the people attending won't know anyone either, so it's an even playing field.

"But what if I don't have any hobbies, Joel? What if I'm not interested in or passionate about anything?"

That's completely okay too, friend. Pick a random group and go. You'll never know if you never go. This reminds me of a time I once flew to Brisbane, spontaneously. It was one of those crazy things I wanted to tick off my bucket list, to fly somewhere within Australia randomly for a day. I woke up one fine morning and thought "this is the day to do it". I wasn't entirely sure where to go, so I drew a map of Australia on a piece of paper. With my eyes closed, I dropped a pen on the paper. It landed on Brisbane. I hopped off the bed, got dressed, picked up my wallet, and headed straight for the airport.

"What can I do for you today?" asked the lady behind the counter.

"I'd like to buy a return ticket to Brisbane, please," I responded.

"Sure, and when would you like to return?" she asked.

"This afternoon, thanks," I said.

"Oh, I see. Are you travelling for business or pleasure?" she asked curiously, though I suspect she already knew the answer, judging by the casual shirt, shorts and flip flops I was wearing.

"Bucket list!" I said triumphantly.

Ha! Good for you," she laughed.

I arrived at Brisbane airport and took the train into the city, feeling expectant. I'd never been to Brisbane before. It felt wild and crazy, but I had a complete ball. Knowing I only had a few hours for this trip, I went straight to the city's main attraction area, South Bank, where I got to see the local museum, the arts centre and Brisbane's iconic man-made beach, called Streets Beach.

I even got to meet new people. It just so happened that there was a classic car meet in the area and I found myself speaking with one of the car owners, a gentleman in his late sixties, with grey hair and a moustache. He asked me where I came from. I told him about my bucket list and that I was heading back to Sydney straight after our conversation. He laughed and grabbed his friends to meet me, asking me to retell my story again. We all had a chuckle and I thoroughly enjoyed learning more about classic cars from these passionate and easy-going enthusiasts. I stayed with the guys for another half an hour and then headed back to the airport. I remember getting home early that night feeling tired but accomplished. Boy, did I have an awesome story to tell my flatmates at the dinner table that evening! But more than that, my trip sparked an interest in me, which later influenced my wife and me to buy a muscle car of our own and join our local Mustang club.

So, give things a go! In the worst-case scenario, it can only add to your life experiences. At best, you might learn something new, find a passion or make new friends.

If you're into exercise, one group that may be of interest is CrossFit, which I talked briefly about in an earlier chapter. Unlike my local gym, CrossFit gyms have a tight community-based system. Let me explain. At a normal gym, you will find people who typically exercise on their own, sometimes with headphones on so you can't talk with them. They don't want to be disturbed; they are there for their own needs. Meanwhile, at a CrossFit studio, people work out together as a group, always helping and pushing each other as a team to get over the line. It's like having your own cheer squad. This wouldn't happen at my local gym. No one would clap for you when you finish a workout! That would seem weird there, quite frankly. To top it off, when I visited, the CrossFit coach and his teammates threw a free barbecue sizzle for everyone afterwards at the park nearby, to help us get to know each other better. Though it's a bit expensive for me, I now understand why people go to CrossFit. Community is a big factor that makes their style of gym a success and it's partly what makes people go back for more. Their camaraderie and support system can help many to achieve the fitness goals they could only dream of reaching on their own. Doing exercise together is also a lot more fun than doing it alone, so I want to encourage you to consider joining a fitness group, whatever that may be (yoga or Pilates, perhaps). You might meet a friend for life or, as in the case of the story below, a life partner.

Perhaps being in the gym doesn't sound like your kind of place to build community—that's completely fine too. Another incredibly fun way to keep fit and meet people is dancing. There are *plenty* of people who (despite a lack of limb coordination) take it up and enjoy themselves. Many years ago, I encouraged one of my best friends, Alan (an expat from the US), to take up salsa lessons with me at a community hall in Redfern that was run by friends of mine from church. One of the great things I found about salsa lessons—apart from learning how to dance, of course—was how quickly you get to meet people. We generally started the lesson paired with a partner, then lined up to form one or more large dance circles. The person on the outside would lead and the person inside would follow. Every thirty seconds or so, the salsa teacher would shout "change" and we would swap partners with the next person in the circle. The class got to know one another very quickly this way. It was almost like going to a speed dating event, only we had to move our bodies, not our mouths (except for all the laughter)!

For Alan, however, it did turn out to be a speed date of sorts. Week after week, he would dance with a beautiful young woman who had the wildest flame-red curls and a strong Kiwi accent. Knowing Alan was single, I decided to see if I could pair the two of them together—a little more permanently. "Hey, Alan, that girl over there with the fiery red hair—she's Danelle. She's originally from New Zealand. I think you should ask her out," I said, egging Alan on, who looked over at her and giggled.

"Yeah, wow. She's pretty but I don't know if I'd be her type," he responded.

"We'll see about that. Let me introduce you to her," I said confidently.

"Okay," Alan replied tentatively.

During a break, I found my window of opportunity and introduced Alan to Danelle, and they hit it off immediately. They went on several dates and if I'm permitted to say, for a moment I didn't think it was going to work out when Alan told me they each paid for their own meals on the first date. Nevertheless, Alan and Danelle are now happily married with a beautiful daughter. And to think this love story may never have happened had Alan chosen not to come along with me to salsa in the first place. In fact, he almost didn't, after telling me he had two left feet!

Challenge time: Can you think of a social group you could give a try this week? Write down a few ideas, some related to your interests and maybe a wild card or two in addition. Apart from Meetup.com, you can also search for groups on LinkedIn if you're more interested in professional groups, or Facebook with its many public groups you can peruse and join.

2. FIND A CAUSE AND VOLUNTEER

Volunteering has become a global movement. Many professionals, seniors, teens and even children are volunteering everywhere to help make the world a better place. Volunteering your time and skills is an excellent way to meet people from all sorts of backgrounds, learn from the life experiences of fellow volunteers and form strong bonds. If you volunteer in your community, you also help to strengthen your community. For example, being part of the Neighbourhood Watch can help reduce crime in the area.

Volunteering can also help you learn all sorts of transferable skills such as leadership, communication and people skills, which are all important life skills to have.

One of the greatest examples I've heard about volunteering is that of former Senior Australian of the Year, David Bussau, a softly spoken man my wife and I had the honour of meeting through a common friend of ours. Back in 1974, David, in his mid-thirties at the time, travelled with his young family to Darwin in the Northern Territory of Australia, after seeing the destruction of the city by tropical Cyclone Tracy on television. With his skills in construction, David headed up a movement by taking a volunteer construction team to help rebuild the city. In his book, *Don't Look Back*, David tells how after having a career in building successful businesses, he began to reassess his life and how to best utilise his time and resources going forward. It was at this time that Cyclone Tracy had devastated the city of Darwin. David felt compelled to answer this call for help. He found a new sense of purpose. David spoke with his wife, Carol, about his new calling and she was more than happy to oblige and support him. David then went to his office and told his construction employees that he was heading to Darwin for an unspecified time and asked if anyone would be interested in joining his cause, to use their skills and help the victims of Cyclone Tracy. There would be no wage, but David would pay for their flights and the necessary tools to bring with them. Rebuilding the city was a challenging but rewarding experience for all who were involved.

That was the first of a series of events that would lead David to devote his life to solving poverty worldwide by becoming a pioneer of microfinance. Together with a colleague, he co-founded Opportunity International, which today has provided micro-loans to over one million people across the world who have lacked access to banks to start a small business.

David is the recipient of many accolades and awards for his work over the past few decades, and I feel privileged and inspired to know him. Despite all he has achieved, David is incredibly humble, quiet and reserved, but his eyes will tell a different story—they give a glimpse into his wisdom, passion and purpose.

Now, I'm not saying we should all start quitting our day jobs and follow in David's footsteps. His story is somewhat unique and truly inspirational, yes. But there are other ways of volunteering our spare time, even by starting out small.

Two years ago, my father-in-law, Mark, retired from work. He wondered what was next for him, so he decided to become a volunteer firefighter with the New South Wales Rural Fire Service, where he received training and eventually became a bushfire and village firefighter. Mark shared with me how one of the first callouts he received was a pager call from the station. A truck had overturned—it was showtime. He remembers the adrenaline rush as they were told a man was trapped inside the vehicle. "Thoughts were running through my head. I was thinking of the possible scenarios that may unfold when we got there, and what we would then need to do to rescue the man out," Mark explained.

Fortunately, by the time they arrived at the scene, both the passenger and driver had managed to get themselves out of the truck on their own, unscathed except for a few minor bruises and cuts.

"Glad to hear!" I exclaimed. "So what was your reason for joining the fire service, Mark?" I asked.

"One of the reasons was to serve the community where there's a need. I get there [at the station] half an hour early to chat with the guys, so there's a social side to it. Some of the younger guys have made friends out of it, too, and turn up to parties whenever they got an invite. For me, however, I enjoy meeting the local community. When we're preparing for bushfire season, we go to the local shopping centre and speak with people, and the kids like to get inside the truck. It all helps to establish rapport with the community. In a sense, it's a newfound purpose after retirement, which means I'm not stuck at home getting bored and wasting away. It helps with my mental health."

If by now you're thinking "I want to volunteer but don't know where to begin", here are some ideas to get the juices flowing:

GET INVOLVED AT A LOCAL SCHOOL

Many schools welcome help from people, whether it be with reading, numeracy, gardening, sports, breakfast or barbecue activities. There could be a role that suits you and your lifestyle.

VOLUNTEER SWIM OR SURF LIFESAVER

You can be an active patrol member saving lives at a local swimming pool or the beach. There are junior activities that introduce children to surf lifesaving, right through to more senior patrol and rescue volunteer roles. If you've ever watched the show Bondi Rescue and think "yeah, I can do that", why not contact your local beach club and ask them about the many ways you can get involved, provided you have the proper skills and training, of course.

NATIONAL PARKS AND WILDLIFE VOLUNTEER

If you've got a passion for nature, maybe you can give this option a try. Not only are the great outdoors peaceful and good for mindfulness, but you'll also get to meet like-minded people. From gardening to weeding, right through to caring for animals, there are plenty of opportunities to help look after our environment.

SOUP KITCHENS AND FOOD RESCUE ORGANISATIONS

There could be dozens of soup kitchens or food vans around your city, run by not-for-profit organisations, which serve underprivileged or homeless individuals. Many of them require volunteers, whether it's to help with fundraising, source food or serve the homeless at a local kitchen. My brother, Erick, used to take his two kids with him every weekend when they were younger, collecting unsold bread from a local bakery and distributing it to families in need. Erick used their volunteering experience to teach his kids about what life is like for the less privileged and to learn the importance of sharing and making a difference to others.

CHARITY AND HUMANITARIAN ORGANISATIONS

In my early twenties, I volunteered in a communications role for the Australian Red Cross in Melbourne, by liaising with and providing support to attendees during volunteer information open days. Apart from the obvious reason of wanting to help others, I also wanted to add to my work experience and improve my ability to communicate effectively with people. It was my first taste of volunteering and it was a great way for me to meet people from all walks of life. There are many other charities out there for you to choose from, so do your research and think about the causes that interest you. Consider your skills, passions and desires before volunteering. The closer the match, the more satisfying and meaningful your volunteering experience will be.

COACHING AND MENTORING

If you are an expert in a particular field, then maybe coaching is for you as a way of giving back. Coaching allows you to help others improve their performance or skills, whether it be at work, sports or something else. Maybe you're great at playing the piano—perhaps you can volunteer your skills in this area and coach the next generation of pianists.

Or perhaps mentoring is more aligned with what you want to do, especially if you've done a bit of living already and would like to build someone else's development in their career, emotional maturity and character. Mentoring is more of a long-term relationship with your protégé. I am grateful and privileged to have had several mentors throughout my adult life who've helped to shape who I am today. So, if you're in a place where you can mentor and bless others, I promise you that your efforts will not go to waste. It's one of the most powerful ways to positively impact someone's life and the spheres they go on to influence. Often, mentors and mentees become friends for life. If you look at all the great leaders of the world, even presidents have coaches and mentors. With your help, someone out there could become the next leader who changes the world for the better.

VOLUNTEER DAD FOR FATHERLESS BOYS

It is a fact that boys develop more courage and confidence in their lives when they have a positive male role model to learn from. If you're a father and this is something close to your heart, perhaps volunteering in this area is something worth looking into.

MIGRANT AND REFUGEE SERVICES

Back in 1991, when we first migrated to Australia from the Philippines, my father, Lito, couldn't find a job, so he volunteered his time at the local migrant resource centre in the western suburbs of Melbourne. Lito, who was a barrister before migrating, had started his professional career as an accountant for a trucking company. Accounting was the skill he was able to leverage to meet a need, which was greatly appreciated by the migrant centre.

If volunteering in migrant and refugee services is something that might interest you, there are many other ways you can provide support and make people feel welcome— not just to newly arrived immigrants, but to asylum seekers, refugees and other people who are vulnerable or perhaps feeling isolated as a result of their migration. Perhaps you might be interested to learn from other cultures and share about ours to help them settle in. I believe that our communities will greatly benefit if we help newcomers settle into our Australian way of life. Speak with your local city council and ask how you can volunteer. It could be as simple as helping someone improve their English through teaching English as a second language (ELS) classes or offering to show them around the neighbourhood—where the grocery stores, library and schools are. You might even volunteer to check in on them occasionally and offer your company. One of the worst things new migrants face is the lack of social contact, which can lead to isolation, loneliness and depression. A simple call or visit can certainly go a long way in boosting their mental health and confidence. The sooner we empower them, the sooner they can transition and contribute to our community.

BUILD A HOME IN POORER NATIONS

Due to poverty, millions of people in the world either lack adequate housing or are homeless. If helping people to have a safe and decent place to live interests you, an organisation that comes to mind is Habitat for Humanity. They are an international not-for-profit organisation with a community of over 4,000 volunteers who travel to developing countries to build homes, communities and hope. I have friends who have done this in the past and they highly recommend volunteering either here on our own soil or overseas. Yes, it will be challenging and yes, you could be working in the sweltering heat; but the experience you gain, the things you learn and the people you meet will be truly rewarding.

❖ ❖ ❖

I hope that I have given you enough ideas to get the wheels in motion. We have only scratched the surface as to how you can volunteer your time, energy and skills. There are many other notable causes out there that may align better with your interests, such as in the disability and aged care sectors. Both of these demographics are at a very high risk of social isolation.

Challenge time: Is there a cause you have in mind or would like to know more about? Maybe now is the time to do something about it—to do your research, put your hand up and volunteer.

3. HOST AN EVENT

Sometimes, a great way to build community is to host your own event and invite people to it. However, if the thought of planning and preparing for it feels a bit overwhelming, you could start out small. It could be as simple as inviting your closest friends over for coffee or inviting a colleague or two out for after-work drinks. As you get the hang of it, you can increase the number of people you invite along. For example, you might start by asking a dozen friends to meet up at the beach (there's not a lot of preparation needed to sit on the sand, swim and talk). If you're feeling more game, what about hosting a barbecue at a local park for a larger group that includes not only your inner circle of friends but your acquaintances as well (as I described in the diagram I shared earlier)?

I did *exactly* that just recently. After ten years of motorbike riding, I finally hosted my first barbecue for my riding community, most of whom were acquaintances, and others I met for the first time. I notified people a few weeks prior, so they could see my Facebook invite and book it in advance. I then sent reminders and follow-up messages during that time to keep it front of mind. My idea was to have a simple sausage sizzle by the river as an opportunity to eat, speak and build the tribe in a relaxed atmosphere. I expected only a few people to come, but 20 people arrived that Saturday morning, ready for a snag and some socialising. I believe the good turnout was in part due to me investing time in that community prior to hosting the event by participating in online discussions and turning up to ride meets, so they knew who I was, or I was at least familiar to each of them, which was enough for them to accept my invite. The meet-up was a success, not because of how many riders came along but because many of them got to meet each other for the first time. One of the riders even mentioned to me that he was looking for work. I said that I might be able to help him and that I'd be more than happy to forward his details and resume to human resources at my work. It didn't guarantee anything but it was my way of offering support and building a relationship with him. That's what I love about these events—you just never know who you'll meet and the friendships you'll make in the process.

Finally, I believe successful community-building should be inclusive. Where it's appropriate and as far as it's feasible with you, no person should ever feel excluded because of how they look, where they're from or their circumstance. So, if you're thinking about hosting your own get-together, consider inviting people who may be different from you or people you wouldn't normally think to invite. You may just meet a friend for life, and/or at the very least, get the opportunity to broaden your social circles.

Whether you're joining a group, volunteering your time for a cause or hosting an event, let me give you three simple steps to remember to improve your success with meeting people and making new friends.

STEP 1: WALK UP TO SOMEONE AND INTRODUCE YOURSELF

For many of us, this is easier said than done. If this is you, don't worry, you're not the only one. It has taken me a long time to have the courage to take the initiative to introduce myself to people. But the more I do it, the easier it gets.

Here's a scenario: Imagine you were invited to an event by the host, Glen. Try not to cling to Glen all night. Walk around and socialise. Try one of these scripts to start a conversation:
1. Hi, I don't think we've met before. My name is Joel. Glen's a friend of mine. How do you know him?

2. Hi, I'm Joel. Nice to meet you. How did you hear about this event?

Keep your icebreakers short. Also notice how the questions are somewhat open-ended, meaning it's going to require the other person to give more than a simple "yes" or "no" response. They might say that Glen is an old friend from school or that they learned about the event from a colleague they tagged along with.

STEP 2: GET THEM TALKING FIRST

Most people will generally dominate a conversation. Don't be that person. Research shows that only about 10 percent of us listen effectively. We often think we are listening but, really, we can't wait to jump in to tell our story. What works best is when we let the other person talk about themselves first and show a genuine interest in what they have to say. You'll know they're done when they want to stop talking and hear more about you next. Not only will you create a great first impression, but they'll also remember you for making them feel listened to. When we seek first to understand, and when we put ourselves in their shoes and hear their point of view, we begin to build rapport and connect with people. The more you actively listen, the more relaxed the conversation becomes, the less anxious you'll feel and the more memorable you become.

STEP 3: EXCHANGE CONTACT INFORMATION

Caveat: This may not happen every time.
If you've been following these steps correctly, you'll get

to a 'bonus round' where the other person might now like to stay connected with you. Depending on the situation, you might want to exchange phone numbers, business cards, add them on Facebook or Instagram, or connect via LinkedIn. Once you do, message them to thank them for their time. To put the icing on the cake, say something in your message that will let them know you listened to them. For example, if the other person is going on a holiday with their family soon, you could say something like, "Hey Beth, it was great meeting you tonight. Enjoy the trip to Fiji with your husband and the two kids. Until next time!" She'll appreciate it and it'll leave a good lasting impression on her.

❧ ❧ ❧

I mentioned several ideas on how you can build new friendships and connections in this chapter. However, I am sure there are plenty of other ways to build your own personal community. What do you think—have I missed some good or even better ideas? What other suggestions would you include? ❧

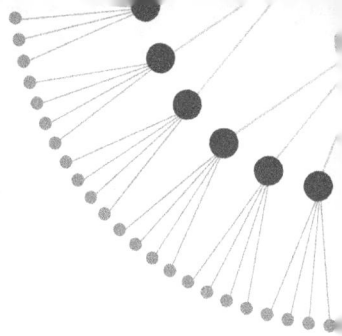

CHAPTER 8

Ways We Can Build a More Connected Society

This final chapter contains tangible ideas for how we can bring connectedness to the forefront of our communities. I believe that tackling and thereby reducing problems associated with loneliness is *everyone's* responsibility and requires all of us to work together—from federal and state governments, councils, leaders, employers, local authorities, health sectors and the general community—to develop and employ initiatives to promote social wellbeing. The following suggestions are nothing new and are not meant to be an exhaustive list—they only scratch the surface. My hope is that these suggestions will spark conversations and generate ideas and action. I would love to hear your thoughts on this subject as well.

CHAT BENCHES

Have you ever sat on a public bench and thought, "I wish I could talk to the person next to me" but felt too awkward to strike up a conversation? What if the seat was a designated chat bench designed for that very purpose? Wouldn't it make it easier to approach strangers then?

I recently ran this idea past Logan's family care educator, Pari, as I was picking him up one day. "Imagine if we could implement 'chat benches' all over Australia," I said. "The idea is simple: when you sit on the public bench, it means you are open for a casual chat with no strings attached. When you're finished talking with the other person, you simply go your separate ways. The idea is to make it easier for people to connect in their local community."

"But what if people take advantage of the vulnerable? How can we avoid that?" Pari asked.

"Perhaps the council needs to make sure these benches are in busy areas where visibility and foot traffic is high. Perhaps chat rules should also be attached on the back of the bench and possibly a contact number for emergency purposes."

Pari smiled and seemed to warm up to the idea. "Oh yes, if I'm not in a rush I could imagine myself sitting down for a chat if I see someone on that seat," she said. "This reminds me, my daughter once told me that in her son's primary school, they have what I think is called a 'buddy bench' in the playground area. When someone sits there, it gives a signal to the other kids that you need social connection. And she told me it works brilliantly. Kids come over or pick up whoever is sitting there and ask them to come and play."

"Wow," I replied, "I've never heard about these buddy benches before. I don't remember seeing them back in the day at any of the schools I went to."

This brief conversation, in a way, helped to validate my idea. If we can have buddy benches in schools, why can't we have chat benches for adults? To make it practical, what if shopping centres and local councils converted some of their existing seats for this purpose? In my local area alone, our village has more than a dozen benches. Can you imagine how many people we could connect in the community if these benches were found in familiar places such as shopping malls, plazas or town centres everywhere?

CHAT TABLES

How many times have you been at a restaurant or café and felt a little uncomfortable about eating on your own? As you sit down and wait for food, you reach straight for your smartphone to look busy. I know this feeling. There are times when I've been happy to eat out by myself, but other times when I wished I had someone to talk to, especially when I'm out of town on business travel. While it was fun to travel in the early years, it began to feel lonely over time. Sometimes I would order dinner and stay inside the hotel room when what I really wished I could do was have a meal in town and explore it with someone like my wife or in the company of friends. While others may say they enjoy their own company, I personally think, for the most part, food tastes so much better when shared in the company of others.

If we can have chat benches in public places, why don't we introduce 'chat tables' too, in venues such as cafés and restaurants? Wouldn't it be nice to have the option of sitting at a chat table when you'd like a bit of social interaction while you eat? Some restaurants have communal tables, which is generally a large table where you can seat more than one group of people at a time. The idea is for diners to socialise with other parties during their lunch or dinner. Each time I've sat at one, however, I never really took the chance to speak with strangers. Rather, I sat there to speak with the person I came with and we politely minded our own business. Those times we did sit at a communal table were because it was the only table available. We had no choice but to sit there. If there was a designated chat table, I think people may feel more comfortable to strike up a conversation with strangers. I'm not suggesting it has to be a big table—venues could use what they already have. Perhaps they could start with one table that can seat at least three people that is clearly marked or reserved as a chat table for people who want to eat and talk with other diners. It may even attract more solo customers who are looking to share a meal at those establishments.

According to the Australian Bureau of Statistics, more than two million Australians live in a single-person house-hold.[1] An article posted by The Canberra Times in May 2019[2] stated that solo dining was on the rise in our capital city, with more than 35,000 of its residents living alone, causing restaurant owners to rethink the way they serve their customers.

When I shared this information with Jade, a colleague of mine who grew up in Canberra, she responded, "Yes, it makes sense—so many venues there are designed to be more approachable for solo diners. Some restaurants, for example, have seats or stools by a bench where you could face the bartender or the chef so you can talk with them".

I said, "That's great. Now imagine adding a chat table so strangers can also strike up a conversation with one another if they wanted. I can only imagine the number of people who travel to Canberra for business reasons. Surely it could make their stay more pleasant and less alone".

"Yes, I would love that idea!" Jade said beaming.

Now, let's think of all the restaurants and cafés one could dine at in Australia. Can you imagine the countless number of people we could connect in the community if these outlets participated in contributing at least one chat table each to this social wellbeing cause? That would be my utopian dream. What do you think?

COMMUNAL SPACES IN NEW HOUSING DEVELOPMENTS

My family and I live in a three-bedroom unit in a block of six apartments, as part of a larger complex. Though I love where we live, I wish it had a communal space with a long dining table where we could eat together with our neighbours every now and then, ask each other how our days were and get to know one another better. Many of the residents here live far away from loved ones—their parents and extended families are either interstate or overseas, especially if they came to Sydney for work (myself included). The neighbours in our complex could sometimes be the closest thing to a family or support network some of us may have. Additionally, many of us can't even see our families due to current travel restrictions. Now, more than ever, it's an important time to build relationships with our neighbours.

The idea for a communal space came from when Belinda and I used to run a weekly connect group in our home. We would welcome five to ten people from our local church over every Tuesday night and pack them into our tiny living room. Sometimes they'd eat before arriving, other times they'd bring food or treats over and have potluck while sharing stories, lessons or discussing the highs and lows of the week, and what we were thankful for. The more we got together, the deeper our relationships became. Once strangers, over time we became close friends, travel buddies, wedding guests and sometimes even the best of lifelong friends as a result. This type of gathering and sharing of life is fantastic and one I'm sure many people wish they could experience in their daily lives. The good news is, it *is* possible if we start building housing developments where the individuals' social wellbeing needs are at the heart of its design.

We can't easily change existing housing developments, but wouldn't it be great if a central communal space was included in brand new apartment complex designs to make them conducive to people coming and eating together in groups? Unfortunately, housing in Australia seems to be more about maximising buyers' private apartment space to deliver the sellers' profit, rather than creating environments that put connection at the centre of their design.

Fortunately, there are developers and other establishments that are challenging the status quo and putting this concept to the test. One such company is WeWork, a provider of shared workspaces for technology start-ups, and now also offers its young professionals a place to stay, called WeLive, in the same building as their offices. Located across two locations in New York and DC, WeLive is a project designed as a co-living space for WeWork residents, complete with community-centric amenities, such as a shared residents' lounge, kitchen, recreational areas and laundry facilities. In a way, it's similar to student living accommodation, but for young professionals.

Jade used to live in a university lodge with 353 individual rooms and similar kinds of communal living benefits and amenities I described at WeLive, including a sizeable rooftop barbeque facility that helped to bring together and connect the resident students.

When I asked Jade whether she made new friends at the lodge as a result of communal living, she responded, "Oh, absolutely. All you had to do was walk into one of the shared rooms and you'd make friends. Everyone was a student and many lived away from home, which is what we had in common. We were all in the same boat and, you could say, needed connection and belonging while living on campus".

But what if you didn't want to live on campus or above your office floor like WeLive but still wanted that urban or inner-city apartment lifestyle with the same co-housing ethos? One particular multi-award-winning apartment building of 24 units in Brunswick, Victoria could be a good starting point. Designed by Breathe Architecture, The Commons was built by a consortium of architects who wanted to create something not only affordable and environmentally sustainable, but with shared facilities such as a communal rooftop space and garden that add a sense of community to its residents, and a ground floor café designed to engage with the broader community. Although this is a great first step for multi-residential housing design in Australia, I believe we could still add more to these features to intentionally connect residents.

In Sweden, there is a large apartment complex called Sällbo (which combines the Swedish words for companionship 'sällskap' and living 'bo'), which houses both the old and young together.[3] Half of the tenants are under the age of 25, while the remainder are pensioners. Sällbo boasts a gym, yoga studio, library, and an arts and crafts studio. It also has a large communal kitchen on every floor. This is a live experiment in intergenerational living by a housing company funded by the city council of Helsingborg, with the primary goal of bringing people together to combat loneliness. A 2019 study found 59 percent of Swedes feel alone often or sometimes.[4] More than half of Swedish homes have a single occupant, which has been attributed to their culture of individualism and a strong welfare state that encourages people to leave home from a young age, so it's common to live alone after leaving school—a trait which continues into old age. In Sällbo however, the young and old are together, and all 72 residents sign a contract promising to spend at least two hours per week with one another. It seems to be working well so far. For example, a 92-year-old former teacher is giving English lessons and, in return, young residents, many of whom are refugees or asylum seekers, help the older residents with technology and social media.

So, what do you think? Could this idea work in Australia? Let's take it up a notch. How about intergenerational living developments where there's retirement living co-located with childcare and a school, with students and young professionals living in the same building or village?

Needing a soundboard for what it would look like to localise these communal space ideas, I reached out to Natalie Pelleri, an old friend and fellow church connect group member, to see if I was heading in the right direction. Natalie is an expert in sustainable environments and urban ecology and has worked for the NSW Government Architects Office. I caught up with Natalie over Zoom to ask about her career with the government.

"Yes, well, after uni, I decided to work at the Architects Office as I wanted to be involved in public projects and work with communities to make people's lives better overall. I did that for over nine years, but now I work with the Inner West Council to increase greening and biodiversity but it's a challenge in these areas," Natalie said.

"I can imagine. That region is already well-built and if I can say, heavily cemented," I added, and she agreed.

"Can you please educate me on what biodiversity is and why it's important for humans?" I asked.

"Sure. Biodiversity is all kinds of trees, plants and birds. There are studies that show having more plant species and greener spaces equates to better mental health outcomes. Humans have this innate need to connect with nature. They feel better, relaxed, refreshed and restored," Natalie explained.

"That makes a lot of sense. We're not meant to be surrounded by these four walls all the time. In my research for this book, I found that we also need to spend more time with nature, where we lived for thousands of years before these man-made walls were built around us."

I went on to share that staying inside for prolonged periods of time can have undesired effects on our health. For example, due to COVID-19 many of us are working remotely but we sometimes forget to take breaks and go for a walk outside. As a result, I for one find that my sleep gets interrupted when I don't get enough sunshine, which is something I'd normally get as I head to work in the morning or when I go on a lunch break. As it happens, there is a strong correlation between the sun and our sleep. In particular, sunlight in the morning triggers our circadian body clock, which helps us to get a good night's rest. As Natalie said, we have this innate need to connect with nature, and for good reason, but we can't do that sitting inside. It's affecting our physical and mental wellbeing, and it's catching many people unaware.

I then wanted to understand from Natalie what the state government has been doing with respect to urban design and social wellbeing.

"A lot of work in the NSW Government right now is beginning to look at the social wellbeing aspect. The Government Architects Office created the 'Practitioner's Guide to Movement and Place'[5], which guides the design and planning around streets and roads and how people experience them but it's more about road networks. The other is they are reviewing the State Environment Planning Policy. Basically, how do we get good design outcomes in our cities and towns? You need to design spaces for the community. I think this one covers your question more broadly," Natalie explained.

"Okay, thanks. That gives me a better context about what the state government is doing at a high level. I'd like to run an idea past you, which is very specific to apartment living and something that local governments could find themselves either championing or falling behind on," I said.

"Please, go ahead," she said inquisitively.

"My utopian dream is to give residents a communal space inside apartment blocks that enables them to intentionally meet and eat together. Imagine coming home from work: you swipe your card to enter the building's main door and the first thing you see is your neighbours right there on the ground floor communal area to greet you. They smile and welcome you by name. The space could have a TV and lounge, a long dining table, maybe a play area for the kids and possibly a couple of office desks. You can use the space to catch up with your neighbours or have meals together. Now, for residents who may not be interested in mingling, there's a back-door entrance, which allows them to get to their apartments easily and under the radar. We can't force people to connect, but we can certainly design places with spaces that enable residents to cross paths and make it more likely for them to stay, talk and gather together. What do you think?"

"I love it! That's a really good idea," Natalie said excitedly, "We have the 'Apartment Design Guide' by the NSW Government, which is a useful tool for councils and developers who are planning residential apartments. Do you know about this guide?"

"Yes, I read it a day ago actually! I understand it talks about basic guidelines to common shared and circulating spaces—such as lobbies, internal corridors and stairs—to provide social and incidental interactions between neighbours, but I feel like the recommendations aren't as intentional about interactions as what I'm envisioning," I replied.

"I hear you. The developers are really the ones to embrace such ideas," Natalie said.

"True, but I feel like it could take forever to convince them, or at least find one willing to think outside the box. Is there anyone in government I can talk to about these things?" I asked.

"Well, yes, there's a Minister of Cities and Urban Infrastructure. You could try approaching them," she said.

"Thanks! You know, the word 'minister' just reminded me, the UK government created the world's first Minister for Loneliness in 2018. It makes me think we should appoint a Minister for Social Wellbeing here in Australia. I don't know why they call them the Minister for Loneliness because 'social wellbeing' sounds more positive and preventative, like something we can work towards rather than something we want to avoid. Anyway, I think a local person in this position could really make a difference in promoting the importance of building deep and meaningful connections and relationships in Australia's society; someone who can permeate all levels of government, business organisations and the community; and someone who is truly passionate about this cause—maybe I should apply for this!" I chuckled.

For further reading, the UK government launched and published a strategic plan, titled 'A connected society: a strategy for tackling loneliness—laying the foundations for change'[6] in October 2018. The publication provides a framework with examples and key pilot initiatives planned by the British government as a call-to-action to help tackle loneliness in the country. It includes everything from social prescribing to teaching the importance of relationships at schools and it contains examples of business and community-led activities, interventions and programs. If you are interested in helping Australia become more socially connected and resilient but don't know where to start, this document is a great launchpad for ideas, and may just give you the inspiration you need.

THE GOOD NEIGHBOUR

I wanted to look at what others have been up to in our community to help combat loneliness when I received an unexpected email from my good friend, Michael McQueen, who wanted to introduce me to a client he had met earlier that morning—the Salvation Army. At the time, they had been working on running a program to address loneliness nationally. Michael told them about me and within hours we had arranged a time to catch up.

It was with great privilege that I met Executive Manager of Innovation, Greig Whittaker, at the Salvation Army (or 'Salvos' as they're commonly known) in Sydney's beautiful Queen Victoria Building. You never know what to expect when you meet people for the first time but Greig was absolutely disarming and so approachable straight off the bat. Wearing his black-rimmed glasses with freshly-cut short hair, Greig quickly went in for a handshake with a big smile.

While we waited for our coffees, I asked Greig to tell me more about the social wellbeing program he was putting together.

"It's called The Good Neighbour, and the program will have three layers: national, local and then individual. First, we'll have a website with a national hotline linking neighbours to neighbours," said Greig. "As an individual, you could phone in from anywhere and we could be having a dialogue. Then we are building it at the local government area. That way we can connect you to someone at a local level, with your neighbour, say, within a 5-kilometre radius.

Once that is done, they can strike up a conversation and go from there. For example, the volunteer neighbour who took the call can say, 'Hey, thanks for chatting with me. Would you like me to buzz you next week?' In a way, we are like a relationship broking service, opening our relational world to others in need and inviting them to that."

"That's a fantastic idea, Greig. As far as I'm aware, I haven't come across anything like this, at least in Australia. I thought this was going to be just another hotline, which is important, but this takes it to another level. How did this idea come about?" I asked.

"Well, since COVID-19, organisations like Lifeline said call rates have gone up but they found that many people are calling really just to have a chat. The Salvos are receiving similar calls, but we don't have a call centre, and we thought, 'Hey if people want someone to talk to then let's find a way to connect them to their own neighbours'. The problem with call centres is you may receive a different operator on the line each time you call. They're not really your friend and the relationship can't go deep. It can also feel traumatic for some people to make them say what they've been through repeatedly to different people. But if we can connect them to people in their neighbourhood who can follow up, be supportive and offer them long-term community, then that could be more helpful, meaningful and sustainable in the long run. That's what a national hotline can't do, is invite you to something," Greg explained.

By that point, I was smiling from ear to ear. I genuinely loved the concept, its great potential to improve people's wellbeing and how it could even save a life. Having experienced this kind of hospitality myself, where good people opened their homes and friendship at a time when I was battling loneliness, I can certainly vouch that it works, at least it did for me.

"So, are you piloting this anywhere, Greig, you know—getting a proof of concept done?" I asked.

"Yes, that's exactly the plan, Joel. For now, we are calling it The Good Neighbour. We're launching it in Ryde next month. We've invited all churches in the area to participate to begin with then we'll on-board anyone who wants to volunteer. We'll have each volunteer police-checked, working with children-checked and trained to be certified volunteers. To create awareness, we are also going to ring every doctor and professional provider in the area and let them know our service is available."

I went home that day with my heart full, knowing that this innovative and much-needed community program was on its way. What I like about the Salvos is that they have a trusted brand and they stand for healthy communities, which makes them well-positioned to get people involved and using this service. Greig and his team have a big task ahead of them, but I know many people will appreciate The Good Neighbour and I am very much looking forward to seeing it become a reality nationally and—with positive results, who knows, even globally.

Another initiative with a similar approach to The Good Neighbour is One Another Community, whose purpose is to encourage people to help each other out, just as good neighbours do. Its founder, Lisa Hollinshead, explained to me how she and several people around the globe banded together to build the website in under three months, with a phone app also on the way. The idea is to post a task you need help with, whether it be buying groceries, walking your dog or simply asking someone to check on you, and you will be connected to a kind and trusted volunteer in your neighbourhood. Unlike Airtasker, where you hire skilled people for a fee, One Another Community is free of charge as it involves people in the community offering their time and skills for a good cause. Naturally, I connected Greig with Lisa, as I believe there could be opportunities for them to collaborate. After all, we're *better together*.

LONELINESS EXHIBITION

I love meeting everyday people doing amazing things to tackle some of humanity's greatest challenges like depression and loneliness. One such individual is Tessa Maree, a freelance filmmaker, writer and storyteller, who in 2019 conducted an immersive street exhibition in London with the aim to reduce the stigma around loneliness and get people talking. My friend Alice Matthews, journalist and host of SBS show *The Feed*, introduced me to Tessa, who wanted to run a similar exhibition in Sydney. Due to the pandemic, Tessa had to return to Australia, but it gave us the opportunity to catch up in person to talk about her work.

Tessa, who I surmised was in her late twenties, caught the train into town from Wollongong. We then sat down at a coffee shop at the QVB and I bought lunch as a small way of saying thanks for making the long trip to Sydney. I was curious to know what inspired Tessa to create a loneliness exhibition, and in London of all places, so that was the first thing I asked.

"When I went to the UK, I was depressed (being far away from home and my friends) and struggled with my own mental health. At the time, I was exploring some topics to do a documentary on. Then, one day, one of our friends took his own life. Hearing how he lost his life to suicide, I realised we are not talking about this topic enough, which is tragic. So, I started working on a short documentary, interviewing five people on their experience with suicide and depression. I was then invited to check out this program at The Loneliness Lab in London. Funded by Lendlease, they wanted to find out if our built-up environments contributed to loneliness. Architects and creatives alike banded together to come up with solutions. While I was there, I met this photographer and together we thought, 'What would happen if we put some photographs and stories into the streets? How would people respond to the issue of loneliness?' So we tested it. We had everyone from students and professionals to the elderly and the homeless, listening, talking and writing down their stories. We then pitched it to the local government, got the funding, and it became an exhibition series," Tessa explained.

"Wow, that's a great story, Tessa. So what did this project teach you about loneliness?" I asked.

"I learned it isn't just about social isolation. For some, it has nothing to do with that. It's more about the disconnect from sense of self, and not knowing who they are on the inside. The knock-on effect is you become socially isolated. The project also showed that if you provide the space, people will open up. Ninety percent of those we surveyed who spoke up about their loneliness had never opened up about it before. I asked questions like, 'What does loneliness feel like to you?' and one guy described it like he was reaching out his arms as wide as he could, but nobody was within reach. Another woman said, 'I'm so full but I have no one to share the fullness with'. Still, another lady described loneliness like being on stage, but with all the lights going out."

While hearing of their experiences through Tessa, I couldn't help but feel their pain. I don't need to imagine it, as I know only too well what those feelings are like.

Tessa and her photographer interviewed 35 people overall, in addition to reviewing hundreds of online submissions, but she'd wanted to talk with more people. Unfortunately, COVID-19 meant the project was put on hold and Tessa decided to return home to Australia to protect her own sense of belonging. She then applied for local government funding to run a similar loneliness exhibition in Sydney but missed out. Nevertheless, I think her idea is thought-provoking, novel and causes people to stop and think; one that sheds light on a predominantly hidden and shadowy topic. I also hope she finds the space and funding to exhibit, despite missing out the first time.

Now that you have read some ideas in this chapter, can *you* think of other creative ways we can help to combat loneliness and build a more aware and connected society in the process? I would love to hear them.

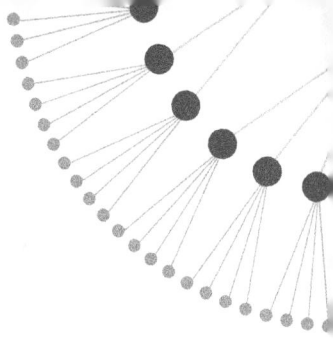

Conclusion

It has been three long years since I began *Better Together* and I never thought it would take this long to not only share my story but source and weave in the most relevant, eye-opening evidence to enrich my narrative. I didn't want to rush things because I know the topic of loneliness, as it relates to our social wellbeing, is very important, so I wanted it to be as well thought out as possible. I also feel it's largely neglected, as most of the focus in mainstream media has been about 'depression' and 'mental health'. Yet despite our efforts to raise awareness about them, depression is *still* an ever-increasing problem all over the world. As I looked closely at my initial research over the years, the more I noticed an underlying theme that was just too significant to ignore: the lack of meaningful relationships and social bonds in our lives are the cause for a lot of mental health problems in our society. Knowing this, I wanted to address loneliness at a deeper level and felt it was the right time to bring social wellbeing to everyone's attention, speak with the experts, get the data and unpack it, then share the findings with as many people as I could, so that together, *we can all be part of the solution.*

To an extent, perhaps I should be somehow thankful for all the horrible and lonely experiences I had growing up, shouldn't I? I mean, they gave me the perspective I needed to see both sides of the coin: firstly, to know what it's like to feel disconnected from supportive and meaningful relationships and how that can lead to a cascade of unwanted physical and mental health issues including severe depression; and secondly, to know what it's like to come out the other end, establishing and nurturing quality friendships that have made a positive impact in my life.

But what if I could go back in time and speak with my younger self as I suffered from chronic loneliness. What would I say to him and where would I meet him? I would probably choose that time I was on the train on my way to university where I felt completely alone in the world, suffocating and unable to physically breathe, wondering if anyone would come and rescue me from my misery. I would come and take a seat next to him. At first, I would say, "You are not alone" and offer him a shoulder to cry on and, for a while, I would just sit there quietly and let him cry it out until he felt calmer and more ready to listen. And then these are the things I would want to tell him:

"Joel, I completely understand what you're going through. It is a very painful experience. But just so you know, you shouldn't blame yourself or feel worthless. There is nothing wrong with you and what you're feeling is completely understandable. We are social beings and, akin to drinking when we are thirsty or eating when we're hungry, when we feel lonely, that's our body's way of reminding us we need social contact. It's hard-wired in all of us, which is why we are all prone to feeling lonely. None of us are immune to it. Our race has survived for hundreds of thousands of years by living physically together with daily face-to-face contact. So, when we feel lonely and disconnected from our friends, our loved ones or the community we live in, that is when our minds start to play tricks on us. Loneliness can even wreak havoc on our thoughts, behaviours and bodies when it persists and becomes chronic. I should know. I have been there and it was debilitating to the point where I couldn't get out of bed anymore.

"What I'm trying to say is 'I'm sorry'. What you're feeling sucks. But I promise you, your world is not about to end here. In fact, it's just the beginning and your future relationships will get deeper and

better. Many years from now, you'll be a completely different person with a more positive outlook on life, where your connections bring joy and make you feel like you belong. You get there eventually when you start building a personal community and surround yourself with a support network filled with a diverse group of friends. I know you find this hard to believe right now, but it will happen. You made it happen. But getting there is not going to be easy. It takes time and effort to nurture rela-tionships, but it's going to be worth it in the end. Some friends you will keep, some you'll let go of, but it's all part of life's journey. Slowly but surely, your social anxiety and low self-esteem will begin to change also. You become more confident and feel alive again, more hopeful and happier because even though life throws you challenges, big and small, you will at least know you're not facing them alone anymore. You have people who love you and have your back. And that is why I know you'll be okay."

Just thinking through the above scenario, wouldn't it be great if every human being on the planet had someone they can call upon, someone they can talk to, someone who can be there in times of need? Unfortunately, many of us don't even feel like we have that one friend or confidant who can sit beside us and listen. You might already have someone in mind who you suspect needs support. It might even include ... you? Despite Australia being one of the wealthiest nations on the planet, so many of us secretly and quietly hide the fact we are feeling lonely or socially isolated, and this will only continue to increase unless we speak up and do something about it. As social beings, our basic and most intrinsic human need—apart from food and water—is having meaningful relationships in order to lead healthier, longer and fuller lives. So why do we allow ourselves to live with loneliness and ignore it? Do we ignore our thirst and hunger? No, we don't. Neither should we ignore loneliness or we'll suffer its harmful consequences.

In this book, I talked about the damaging, catastrophic effects loneliness can have on our minds and bodies, and I shared some ways we can build new connections to tackle these effects. However, this book was never intended to be the silver bullet to solving loneliness. Rather, my intention was to bring awareness to the subject, so we can come together and find sustainable ways to prevent mental ill-health due to loneliness from happening in the first place. It wouldn't surprise me if depression figures were to decrease as a consequence of such efforts. When people feel connected, supported and as though they belong, the healthier and happier they will be. This can only result in us having a more prosperous and resilient country.

I want to experience a world where children are close to their parents and feel they can discuss just about anything; where young people don't have to succumb to peer pressure because they have solid, healthy relationships; where marriages are richer; where businesses put emphasis on the wellbeing of their employees; where migrants feel accepted;

where minorities feel heard and included; where intergenerational relationships are strong; where older people feel respected and not forgotten; and where *all* people feel they are part of and supported by their community. This is my utopian dream, but I'm sure many others would dream of this also.

For my international readers, I hope you found this book useful. Even though much of the content is localised for Australia, I believe many of the facts and stories told here are universal in nature. After all, we may be separated by land but we are all human citizens of this planet in need of human contact. May this book encourage you to build deep and meaningful relationships and help you to spread the importance of social wellbeing in your region of the world. The sooner we create awareness, the sooner we can advance change. Our survival depends on it.

And remember, no one should ever have to go through life alone. As a species, we truly are—***Better Together.*** ✤

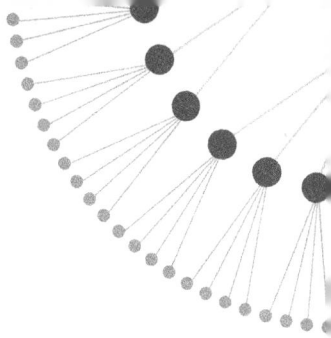

Acknowledgments

Firstly, I'd like to take this opportunity to thank my wife, Belinda, for supporting and encouraging me to write this book and for the countless conversations we spent discussing my thoughts and ideas—often at the dinner table—and challenging me about them at the same time. I believe every writer should have a soundboard and I was glad to have her by my side. I've also been blessed by Belinda's academic background. With a PhD in neuroscience, not only was she helpful when it came to uncovering the inner workings of the brain and our human physiology, but her analytic mind was also a great asset: she didn't just accept my simple explanation of how things worked, but insisted I both build and unpack the evidence and explain the significance of my findings. Belinda sanity-checked my entire manuscript through each draft. She was here copyediting and proof-reading my book along the way. Being an author herself, her experience helped me immensely throughout the entire process, from book writing to publishing to printing and delivery. If you're interested to know more about Belinda and her published book, *Wildflowers*, which shares the stories and photography of survivors of human trafficking, go to www.belindaramirez.net.

I also want to thank my friend, international speaker and prolific author, Michael McQueen, for taking interest in my book and challenging me to refine and narrow my focus from mental health more broadly, to loneliness, a topic where I could easily share my story; and for helping me believe that it's the right subject, the right time and that I'm the right person to talk about it. Thank you, Michael—you've helped me to shed light on what's been a largely ignored but incredibly important topic. Michael also suggested the title, *Better Together*, during our conversation in his living room! Calling this man a friend for the past ten years has been a huge blessing for me. For those interested in Michael's work, go to www.michaelmcqueen.net.

Allison Hiew was my developmental editor, helping me reshape the structure and flow of *Better Together*. She challenged the way I navigated the plot, with the goal of helping me create the best possible experience for my readers and give me the best chance of imparting my message with maximum effect. I hope I have done your work justice, Allison.

My cover design was done by the exceptionally talented Liz Knapp from Mezzanine Media. I wanted to illustrate the circle of friends a person can build for themselves, while positioning one lonely dot disconnected from the rest of its community. Liz understood the essence of what I wanted to convey and the result is this book's beautiful cover. Thank you, Liz.

A huge thanks to all the doctors, psychologists and experts in the field I interviewed for the book including Dr Michelle Lim, Dr Brock Bastian, David Morley, Dr Bethan Richards and Dr Zoya Jamshidi. I really appreciate all of your invaluable time, wisdom and insight. I would also like to thank the rest of the people who shared their stories for this book, as well as the other authors whose works I referred to throughout this book, such as the late Dr John T. Cacioppo. It is possible that my thoughts and ideas may differ from how each of these individuals intended to express or view certain ideas. So, any error of interpretation in this book is my complete responsibility. If you happen to find any, please message me via my website, joelramirez.net and I'll be sure to make any corrections for future editions and reprints of the book.

Thank you also to Graeme Cowan for writing this book's foreword. I sincerely appreciate your input into this subject and for recommending it to my readers.

I want to thank John Munnelly at KPMG (aka 'Chief') for allowing me to work part-time so I could invest some regular and consistent effort into writing this book. And thank you to my team at Wiise.com for supporting me on this journey also.

If anyone is looking for a copyeditor, I'd highly recommend Lisa Ndeira from Write Way Australia. Both my wife and I have now used her manuscript editing services and they have been nothing short of outstanding. Amy Galliford helped format my references, while Julie Hodgins in the US was my typesetter.

A very special mention goes to my parents, Lito and Cora, as well as my brothers, Erick and Francis, my aunt Amelia (Tita Mel), my uncle Adelio (Tito Deo) and family friend, Eric Chan, who were all there for me when I went through loneliness and depression. Thank you all so much for being my faithful family and friends, and keeping me company when I needed it the most.

And finally, to all of my friends, including Alan Bronowicz, Heather Neighbors, Matthew Ng, Billy Adhi, Matt Ketcher, Simon Wu and many, many others—you know who you are—for always being there for me, believing in me, supporting me, encouraging me, challenging me and doing life with me. You are the reason why this book exists. You're *my* dots, *my* better together. Thank you for making me feel like I belong, like I can do anything, and for choosing to be my friend. You are why my faith in humanity is restored, revived and refreshed on a daily basis.

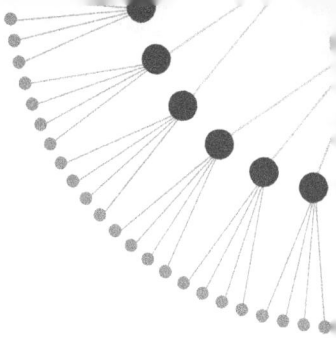

Resources

Please note: the following is not an exhaustive list but rather a starting point for educational purposes or for those seeking wellbeing assistance. If in doubt, speak with your local general practitioner for advice. Otherwise, if the matter is urgent or life threatening, contact 000 immediately.

EMERGENCY CONTACTS

000 EMERGENCY

000

If you are in an emergency situation or need immediate assistance.

LIFELINE

www.lifeline.org.au • 13 11 14

Provides all Australians access to crisis support
and suicide prevention services.

KIDS HELPLINE

www.kidshelpline.com.au • 1800 55 1800

Free 24/7 phone and online counselling service for young people.

1800RESPECT

www.1800respect.org.au • 1800 737 732

Support if you, or someone you know, is experiencing
sexual assault or domestic and family violence.

SUICIDE CALL BACK SERVICE

www.suicidecallbackservice.org.au • 1300 659 467

Provides immediate telephone counselling
and support in crisis for ages 15+.

ORGANISATIONS FOCUSED ON SOCIAL WELLBEING

FRIENDS FOR GOOD

www.friendsforgood.org.au

A volunteer-driven not-for-profit and Australian loneliness pioneer.

FRIENDLINE

www.friendline.org.au

For anyone who needs to reconnect or just wants a chat.
All conversations are casual and anonymous.

NEIGHBOURHOOD CONNECT

www.neighbourhoodconnect.org.au

A national charity and not-for-profit community organisation,
helping people connect with others who live near them.

ENDING LONELINESS TOGETHER

www.endingloneliness.com.au • *02 9339 6001*

A national network of organisations partnering to address the
growing problem of loneliness in people living in Australia.

RELATIONSHIPS AUSTRALIA

www.relationships.org.au • *1300 364 277*

A non-profit provider of relationship support services
for individuals, families and communities.

AUSTRALIAN MEN'S SHED ASSOCIATION

www.mensshed.org • *1300 550 009*

Men's sheds provide a place where men can feel included and safe.
Their aim is to improve the health and wellbeing of their members.

MENTAL HEALTH ORGANISATIONS

HEADSPACE

www.headspace.org.au • 1800 650 890

Provides free online and telephone support and counselling to young people aged 12 to 25 and their families and friends.

BEYOND BLUE

www.beyondblue.org.au • 1300 22 4636

A mental health and wellbeing support organisation. They provide support programs to address issues related to depression, suicide, anxiety disorders and other related mental illnesses.

QLIFE

www.qlife.org.au • 1800 184 527

Provides Australia-wide anonymous LGBTI peer support and referral for people wanting to talk about a range of issues including sexuality, identity, gender, bodies, feelings or relationships.

MENSLINE

www.mensline.org.au • 1300 78 99 78

National telephone and online support, information and referral service for men with family and relationship concerns.

REACHOUT.COM

www.reachout.com • 02 8029 7777

An internet service for young people that provides information, support and resources about mental health issues and enables them to develop resilience, increase coping skills, and facilitate help-seeking behaviour.

OTHER ORGANISATIONS

RU OK?

www.ruok.org.au • www.ruok.org.au/contact

A non-profit suicide prevention organisation. It revolves around the slogan 'R U OK?', and advocates for people to have conversations with others.

THE BLACK DOG INSTITUTE

www.blackdoginstitute.org.au • 02 9382 4530

A non-profit facility for diagnosis, treatment and prevention of mood disorders such as depression, anxiety and bipolar disorder.

SANE AUSTRALIA

www.sane.org • 1800 18 7263

A national mental health charity that offers services to support all Australians affected by complex mental health issues.

CARERS AUSTRALIA

www.carersaustralia.com.au • 1800 422 737

Advocates and lobbies on a wide range of issues that affect carers and also manages the delivery of national programs, support and services for carers across Australia.

WAYAHEAD

www.wayahead.org.au • 1300 794 991

Educates people about mental health and supports them to improve their wellbeing.

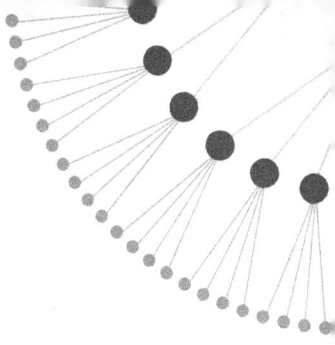

References

CHAPTER 2

1. Bastian B. Shared pain brings people together. *Association for Psychological Science*. 9 September, 2014. https://www.psychologicalscience.org/news/releases/shared-pain-brings-people-together.html

CHAPTER 3

1. De Neve JE, Krekel C. Cities and happiness: A Global Ranking and Analysis. *World Happiness Report*. 20 March, 2020. https://worldhappiness.report/ed/2020/cities-and-happiness-a-global-ranking-and-analysis/

2. Babington B. Loneliness: a growing national challenge. *Families Australia*. 30 January, 2018. https://familiesaustralia.org.au/loneliness-a-growing-national-policy-challenge/

3. Australian Psychological Society, Swinburne University of Technology. Australian loneliness report. Psychology Week. November, 2018.

4. Jennings-Edquist G. Feeling isolated? You're not alone. Here's why 1 in 4 of us is lonely. *ABC Everyday*. 16 November, 2018. Updated 16 December, 2018. https://www.abc.net.au/everyday/social-isolation-why-are-we-so-lonely/10493414

5. Hofstede Insights. What about Australia?. *Hofstede Insights*. 2021. https://www.hofstede-insights.com/country/australia/

CHAPTER 4

1. Collins Dictionary. Definition of 'loneliness'. Collins Dictionary. 2021. https://www.collinsdictionary.com/dictionary/english/loneliness

2. Lifeline. Loneliness and isolation. *Lifeline*. 2021. https://www.lifeline.org.au/get-help/information-and-support/loneliness-and-isolation/

3. Cacioppo JT, Patrick W. *Loneliness: Human Nature and the Need for Social Connection*. W. W. Norton & Company; 2008; 7.

4. Cirino E. What Are the Benefits of Hugging?. *Healthline*. Updated 11 April, 2018. https://www.healthline.com/health/hugging-benefits

5. Cacioppo. *Loneliness*. 14.

6. Cacioppo. *Loneliness*. 17.

7. Cacioppo JT, Hawkley LC, Ernst JM, Burleson M, Berntson GG, Nouriani B, Spiegel D. Loneliness within a nomological net: An evolutionary perspective. *Journal of Research in Personality*. 2006 (40): 1068. DOI: 10.1016/j.jrp.2005.11.007

8. Cacioppo. *Loneliness*. 87.

9. Cacioppo. *Loneliness*. 88.

10. Twenge JM, Ciarocco NJ, Baumeister RF, DeWall CN, Bartels JM. Social Exclusion Decreases Prosocial Behavior. *Journal of Personality and Social Psychology*. 2007; 92 (1): 56. DOI: 10.1037/0022-3514.92.1.56

11. Twenge et. al. Social Exclusion. 59.

12. Cacioppo. *Loneliness*. 32.

13. Cacioppo. *Loneliness*. 108.

14. Celmer L. Partial sleep deprivation linked to biological aging in older adults. *American Academy of Sleep Medicine*. 10 June, 2015. https://aasm.org/partial-sleep-deprivation-linked-to-biological-aging-in-older-adults/

15. Berkman LF, Syme SL. Social networks, host resistance, and mortality: a nine-year follow-up study of Alameda County residents. *American Journal of Epidemiology*. 1979; 109 (2): 186-204. https://doi.org/10.1093/oxfordjournals.aje.a112674

16. Cacioppo. *Loneliness*. 93.

17. Cacioppo. *Loneliness*. 105.

18. Pressman SD, Cohen S, Miller GE, Barkin A, Rabin RS, Treanor JJ. Loneliness, social network size, and immune response to influenza vaccination in college freshmen. *Health Psychology*. 2005 (3): 297-306. DOI: 10.1037/0278-6133.24.3.297

19. Fetters A. What loneliness does to the human body. *Special Broadcasting Service*. 23 January, 2018. https://www.sbs.com.au/topics/voices/health/article/2018/01/23/what-loneliness-does-human-body

20. Cacioppo. *Loneliness*. 106.

21. Cacioppo. *Loneliness*. 106.

22. Hermes GL, Delgado B, Tretiakova M, Cavigelli SN, Krausz T, Conzen SD, McClintock MK. Social isolation dysregulates endocrine and behavioral stress while increasing malignant burden of spontaneous mammary tumors. *PNAS*. 2009; 106 (52): 22393-22398.

23. Reynolds P, Kaplan G. Social connections and risk for cancer: prospective evidence from the Alameda County study. *Behavioral Medicine.* 1990; 16 (3): 101-110. https://doi.org/1 0.1080/08964289.1990.9934597

24. Fleisch Marcus A, Illescas AH, Hohl BC, Llanos AAM. Relationships between social isolation, neighborhood poverty, and cancer mortality in a population-based study of US adults. *PLOS ONE.* 2017; 12(3): e0173370. https://doi.org/10.1371/ journal.pone.0173370

25. Holt-Lunstad J, Smith TB, Layton JB. Social relationships and mortality risk: a meta-analytic review. *PLOS Medicine.* 2010; 7 (7). https://doi.org/10.1371/journal.pmed.1000316

26. Pinker S. The secret to living longer may be your social life. *TED.* April, 2017. https://www.ted.com/talks/susan_ pinker_the_secret_to_living_longer_may_be_your_social_ life?referrer=playlist-what_s_the_secret_to_living_longer

27. Sutin AR, Stephan Y, Luchetti M, Terracciano A. Loneliness and risk of dementia. *The Journals of Gerontology: Series B.* 2020; 75 (7): 1414–1422. https://doi.org/10.1093/geronb/gby112

28. Courtney AL, Meyer ML. (2020). Self-other representation in the social brain reflects social connection. *Journal of Neuroscience.* 2020; 40 (29): 5616-5627.

29. Tomova L, Wang KL, Thompson T. Matthews GA, Takahashi A, Tye KM, Saxe R. Acute social isolation evokes midbrain craving responses similar to hunger. *Nature Neuroscience.* 2020; 23 (12): 1597-1605. DOI: 10.1038/s41593-020-00742-z

CHAPTER 5

1. Hogenboom M. How did the last Neanderthals live?. *BBC Future.* 30 January, 2020. https://www.bbc.com/future/ article/20200128-how-did-the-last-neanderthals-live

2. Zimmermann KA. Pleistocene Epoch: Facts About the Last Ice Age. *Live Science.* Updated 29 August, 2021. https://www.livescience.com/40311-pleistocene-epoch.html

3. Cacioppo. *Loneliness.* 67.

4. Cacioppo. *Loneliness.* 70.

5. Polack E. New Cigna Study Reveals Loneliness at Epidemic Levels in America. *Cigna.* 2 May, 2018. https://www.cigna.com/about-us/newsroom/news-and-views/press-releases/2018/new-cigna-study-reveals-loneliness-at-epidemic-levels-in-america

6. The facts on loneliness. *Campaign to End Loneliness.* https://www.campaigntoendloneliness.org/the-facts-on-loneliness/

7. European Commission. Loneliness—an unequally shared burden in Europe. *Science for Policy Briefs.* https://ec.europa.eu/jrc/sites/jrcsh/files/fairness_pb2018_loneliness_jrc_i1.pdf

8. Prosser M. Searching for a cure for Japan's loneliness epidemic. *Huffington Post.* 15 August, 2018. https://www.huffingtonpost.com.au/entry/japan-loneliness-aging-robots-technology_n_5b72873ae4b0530743cd04aa?ri18n=true

9. The Japan Times. Going it alone: Solo dwellers will account for 40% of Japan's households by 2040, forecast says. *The Japan Times.* 13 January, 2018. https://www.japantimes.co.jp/news/2018/01/13/national/social-issues/going-alone-solo-dwellers-will-account-40-japans-households-2040-forecast-says/#.XeVbeegzZPZ

10. The Social Report 2016—Te pūrongo oranga tangata. *Ministry of Social Development.* https://socialreport.msd.govt.nz/social-connectedness/loneliness.html

11. World Health Organisation. Depression. *World Health Organisation.* 30 January, 2020. https://www.who.int/news-room/fact-sheets/detail/depression

12. Hawkley LC, Capitano JP. Perceived social isolation, evolutionary fitness and health outcomes: a lifespan approach. *Philosophical Transactions B.* 2015; 370 (1669):20140114 https://doi.org/10.1098/rstb.2014.0114

13. What Makes A Good Relationship?. *Relationships Australia.* 2021. https://www.raq.org.au/article/what-makes-good-relationship

14. Company Info. *Facebook.* 2021. https://about.facebook.com/company-info/

15. Turkle S. *Alone Together—Why We Expect More from Technology and Less from Each Other.* Perseus; 2012; 187.

CHAPTER 6

1. Pinker S. *The Village Effect: Why Face-to-face Contact Matters.* Atlantic Books; 2014; 112.

2. Guang G, Roettger ME, Cai T. The integration of genetic propensities into social-control models of delinquency and violence among male youths. *Biosocial Theories of Crime* 2017; 209-234.

3. Fox M. Study finds genetic link to violence, delinquency. *Reuters.* 15 July, 2008. https://www.reuters.com/article/us-delinquents-genes-idUSN1444872420080714

4. Franko DL, Thompson D, Affenito SG, Barton BA, Striegel-Moore RH. What mediates the relationship between family meals and adolescent health issues. *Health Psychology.* 2008; 27 (2): 109-117. DOI: 10.1037/0278-6133.27.2

5. Harrison ME, Norris ML, Obeid N, Fu M, Weinstangel H, Sampson M. Systematic review of the effects of family meal frequency on psychosocial outcomes in youth. *Can Fam Physician.* 2015; 61 (2): 96-106.

6. Causes of Death, Australia. *Australian Bureau of Statistics*. 23 October, 2020. https://www.abs.gov.au/statistics/health/causes-death/causes-death-australia/latest-release

7. Eglit GML, Palmer BW, Martin AS, Tu X, Jeste DV. Loneliness in schizophrenia: construct clarification, measurement, and clinical relevance. *PLoS One*. 2018; 13 (3). DOI: 10.1371/journal.pone.0194021

8. Migration, Australia. *Australian Bureau of Statistics*. 2021. https://www.abs.gov.au/statistics/people/population/migration-australia/latest-release

9. Marriages and Divorces, Australia. *Australian Bureau of Statistics*. 2019. https://www.abs.gov.au/statistics/people/people-and-communities/marriages-and-divorces-australia/2018

10. Jalili C. Feeling Lonely in Your Relationship? Here's What to Do About It. *Time*. 19 March, 2019. https://time.com/5548386/feeling-lonely-in-relationship/

11. Bruess C. Are you lonely in your partnership or marriage? *Ideas TED*. 7 January, 2020. https://ideas.ted.com/are-you-lonely-in-your-partnership-or-marriage/

12. Relationship problems. *Australian Psychological Society*. 2021. https://www.psychology.org.au/for-the-public/Psychology-topics/Relationship-problems

13. Whisman MA, Uebelacker LA. Impairment and distress associated with relationship discord in a national sample of married or cohabiting adults. *Journal of Family Psychology*. 2006; 20 (3): 369.

14. Smart C. *They'll Be Okay: 15 Conversations to Help Your Child Through Troubled Times*. Hachette Australia; 2019; 11.

15. Smart. *They'll Be Okay*. 10.

16. Smart. *They'll Be Okay*. 13.

17. Smart. *They'll Be Okay*. 16.

18. Workplace Loneliness, 2019, Reventure Ltd., page 8.

19. Strack R. Decoding Global Talent. *Boston Consulting Group*. 6 October, 2014. https://www.bcg.com/en-au/publications/2014/people-organization-human-resources-decoding-global-talent

20. Achor S, Kellerman GR, Reece A, Robichaux A. America's Loneliest Workers, According to Research. *Harvard Business Review*. 19 March, 2018. https://hbr.org/2018/03/americas-loneliest-workers-according-to-research

21. Edelman Intelligence. Freelancing in America: 2017. *Upwork*. 28 September, 2017. https://www.slideshare.net/upwork/freelancing-in-america-2017/1

22. McDonald P, Williams P, Stewart A, Oliver D, Mayes R. Digital Platform Work in Australia Preliminary findings from a national survey. *Analysis & Policy Observatory*. 18 June, 2019.

CHAPTER 7

1. Pinker S. The secret to living longer may be your social life. *TED*. April, 2017. https://www.ted.com/talks/susan_pinker_the_secret_to_living_longer_may_be_your_social_life?referrer=playlist-what_s_the_secret_to_living_longer

CHAPTER 8

1. Household and Family Projections, Australia. *Australian Bureau of Statistics*. 14 March, 2019. https://www.abs.gov.au/statistics/people/population/household-and-family-projections-australia/latest-release

2. Hardy K. Why solo dining is on the rise in Canberra. *The Canberra Times*. 21 May, 2019. https://www.canberratimes.com.au/story/6133924/a-table-just-for-one-the-rise-of-solo-dining/#gsc.tab=0

3. Robertson D. 'It's like family': the Swedish housing experiment designed to cure loneliness. *The Guardian.* 15 September, 2020. https://amp.theguardian.com/world/2020/sep/15/its-like-family-the-swedish-housing-experiment-designed-to-cure-loneliness

4. WSP. Six out of ten Swedes feel lonely - most common among young adults and in larger cities. *WSP.* 5 September, 2019. https://www.wsp.com/sv-SE/nyheter/2019/sex-av-tio-svenskar-kanner-sig-ensamma

5. Government Architect. Practitioner's guide to movement and place. *Implementing Movement and Place in NSW.* March 2020.

6. A connected society. A strategy for tackling loneliness—laying the foundations for change. *Department for Digital, Culture, Media and Sport.* October, 2018.